THE PARENT'S COMPLETE
GUIDE TO AYURVEDA

THE PARENT'S COMPLETE GUIDE TO AYURVEDA

PRINCIPLES, PRACTICES, AND RECIPES FOR HAPPY, HEALTHY KIDS

Jayarajan Kodikannath, BSc, BAMS
Alyson Young Gregory, AHC

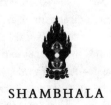

SHAMBHALA

Shambhala Publications, Inc.
2129 13th Street
Boulder, Colorado 80302
www.shambhala.com

Cover art: Elena Kutuzova/iStockphoto; AnnaFrajtova/iStockphoto; and krugli/iStockphoto
Cover design: Katrina Noble
Interior design: Katrina Noble

Disclaimer: This book is a general guide only and is not intended as a substitute for the skill, knowledge, and experience of a qualified medical or mental health professional. The reader should consult a physician before following any of the Ayurvedic recommendations suggested here. The authors, publisher, and their distributors are not responsible for any adverse effects or consequences resulting from the use of the information in this book.

9 8 7 6 5 4 3 2 1

First Edition
Printed in the United States of America

Shambhala Publications makes every effort to print on acid-free, recycled paper.

Shambhala Publications is distributed worldwide by Penguin Random House, Inc., and its subsidiaries.

LIBRARY OF CONGRESS CATALOGING-IN-PUBLICATION DATA
Names: Kodikannath, Jayarajan, author. | Gregory, Alyson Young, author.
Title: The parent's complete guide to Ayurveda: principles, practices, and recipes for
    happy, healthy kids / Jayarajan Kodikannath, BSc, BAMS; Alyson Young Gregory.
Description: Boulder, Colorado: Shambhala, [2022] | Includes index.
Identifiers: LCCN 2021054250 | ISBN 9781611808520 (trade paperback)
Subjects: LCSH: Medicine, Ayurvedic—Popular works. | Self-care, Health—Popular works.
Classification: LCC R605.K63 2022 | DDC 615.5/38—dc23/eng/20211206
LC record available at https://lccn.loc.gov/2021054250

CONTENTS

INTRODUCTION

FROM THE MOMENT a child is born, there is a tender openness that will grow and flourish in direct harmony with the ways they are supported and the spirit with which they are nurtured.

Ayurveda underscores childhood as being the most essential period for shaping and developing a healthy, balanced human being in a person's lifetime, which extraordinarily mirrors the same unconscious, instinctive view of care every parent desires to give their child in support of their physical, mental, and emotional development. Parents intuitively know these are not separate aspects of development, and many are in search of an integrated wellness blueprint that backs them in being fully conscious parents. The principles of Ayurveda are thus more relevant today than ever before.

The Parent's Complete Guide to Ayurveda provides parents with daily lifestyle tools and routines that empower a practical approach to the wellness of their child's body, mind, and spirit. Renowned and beloved scholar of Ayurvedic medicine Dr. Jayarajan Kodikannath explains the step-by-step lifestyle routines and benefits of Ayurveda, allowing the modern-day family to share in individually tailored wellness practices. Dr. J, as he is affectionately known, sets up this first complete guidebook to Ayurveda for children in a most graspable and adaptable way, drawing from decades of clinical experience and earnestly representing a lineage of Ayurvedic practitioners from Kerala, India—Ayurveda's motherland.

Today's parents have the unique ability to endlessly amass information—which often results in feeling overwhelmed and uncertain at times when it comes to making simple lifestyle choices for their families. Dr. J undertakes this unique, collective dilemma of the modern age and addresses parents' everyday questions as well as Ayurvedic perspectives on the critical pandemics of childhood illness in the twenty-first century that parents face today such as ADHD, anxiety, diabetes, and obesity.

So what is Ayurveda? Ayurveda is a natural, holistic life science from ancient India spanning more than five thousand years of history built on natural principles and a philosophy that identifies whole beings and nature as one. Ayurveda considers all aspects of existence including the physical, or structural; the energetic, or functional; and the spiritual, or consciousness—the life within every being. Mind falls under the functional, or energetic, layer of our existence. The Sanskrit term *Ayurveda* comes from two smaller words: *Ayur* meaning "life" and *Veda* meaning "wisdom or science," marking Ayurveda as the science of life and beautifully encompassing the idea of this life as a period of time in which our physical bodies, sense organs, mind, and soul join together for a journey that is perfectly facilitated by nature.

The ancient Ayurvedic texts define this natural, scientific healing system in eight clinical branches: *Kayacikitsa* (general medicine), *Salya Tantra* (surgery), *Shalakya Tantra* (ear, nose, throat, and eye diseases), *Kaumarabhritya* (pediatrics), *Agada Tantra* (toxicology), *Bhuta Vidya* (psychiatry), *Rasayana Tantra* (the science of rejuvenation), and *Vajikarana* (reproductive medicine).

Kaumarabhritya, Sanskrit for "pediatrics," is considered the most important branch and is devoted to supporting the rapid period of growth and development in early childhood that constitutes the building blocks of every child's future as well as an uninterrupted transition to healthy adulthood. The principles of Kaumarabhritya illuminate the ways parents can nurture and maintain positive health for their child both in the present and for the future to ensure a harmonious life whose unique purpose can be fully accomplished. *The Parent's Complete Guide to Ayurveda* clearly explains these principles wholly extracted from the root texts and offers parents guidelines that are both preventive and corrective in nature, focused on children three to sixteen years old.

As Ayurveda gains popularity around the globe, more and more parents are recognizing different ways the guidance and principles resonate with their own inner wisdom, making it a true and valuable companion for every parent's journey regardless of age, race, or circumstance. Much like parenting, the science of Ayurveda is intuitive and profoundly considers the physical, mental, and emotional development of a child as on par with one another. Ayurveda looks carefully at both a child's exposures to external influences and how those inputs are metabolized and expressed for a true view of the whole child. Perfectly in-step with the demands of the modern world, Ayurveda recognizes inputs beyond just diet and lifestyle practices, weighing various sensory stimuli and what is happening on a day-to-day basis in a child's environment as instrumental in influencing their physical, mental, behavioral, and social health and well-being.

Most modern health sciences today focus on the singular dimension of a person's physical body to assess health, whereas Ayurveda honors the uniqueness of every individual's body, mind, and spirit and de-emphasizes the one-size-fits-all approach to wellness. It is the same when it comes to supporting and caring for children. Ayurveda considers the whole child and all the parameters that affect health and development, both directly and indirectly, along with various factors including age, a child's unique nature, and how a child is expressing in the moment to help them grow and develop into their best possible self. The purpose of this book is to guide parents through a series of easy-to-follow tools and markers that allow them to customize diet and lifestyle routines tailored to their child's individual nature as expressed in the mind-body types known as *prakriti*.

What will that look like? While many parenting books tailor specific guidance and advice to different ages and stages of childhood, Ayurveda guides individuals based on their unique nature. This book provides Ayurvedic principles of parenting that you can customize or tailor based on your child's unique needs. Here is what you can expect to learn throughout this book. First, in part one, we'll explore the concept of mind-body consciousness and different ways you can closely observe your child's behavior to gain knowledge of their individual tendencies and needs, as well as identify your child's body constitution along with traditional practices to support them. A quiz in this section will help you identify your child's prakriti. Next, in part two, we'll delve into the four inputs of life central to your child's exposures to the world around them: food, water, breath, and perception. Part three takes us into ways to optimally structure everyday routines and create lifestyle habits that will provide children with a solid foundation to live their best day-to-day life and develop into healthy, harmonious, happy, peaceful adults. Here, we'll cover sleep, activity, and daily routines, as well as ways the traditional Ayurvedic practices of yoga, meditation, and mantras can promote mindfulness, joy, and peace so children can thrive and live a happy, healthy life.

You've surely heard before that *an ounce of prevention is worth a pound of cure*. Emphasis on prevention is a core tenet of Ayurveda, and there is no better time to emphatically focus on prevention than in childhood. The pediatric branch of Ayurveda not only explains how to ensure a child's proper development and growth, it also sets forth principles and natural guidance for prevention and management of various pediatric health problems that can arise due to nutritional and lifestyle imbalances or environmental influences. In addition to seasonal and everyday guidelines, in part four parents will discover the etiology of many disorders according to Ayurvedic principles and learn how to incorporate simple and effective natural herbs and home remedies as both preventive health measures and to ensure the strength and balance of their child's digestive system, immune system, and emotional health.

Children are the future of this world; a million flower buds about to bloom and disperse their fragrance and most pleasing and vibrant impressions to everything and everyone surrounding them. *The Parent's Complete Guide to Ayurveda* is written for every parent and caregiver journeying alongside their child in mind, body, and spirit to nurture the expression of the highest human potential possible during a child's life. It is our hope that the clear understanding and user-friendly format of these various components will help parents to be prepared and proactive in supporting their child throughout this pivotal period of growth and development. Our greatest wish is to empower parents everywhere to grace every child with support of body, mind, and spirit so that they may realize their innate potential and live in joy. We are grateful and humbled by the opportunity to share Dr. J's experiences as a practitioner and transmit the Ayurvedic traditions of his lineage to you and your children.

Note

In this book, we will look at common childhood ailments and disorders as well as how to manage them and the therapeutic interventions recommended by Ayurveda. Please remember traditional therapeutic interventions should always be guided by an Ayurvedic physician, who will personalize treatment for your child based on constitution, age, and stage of the condition or disorder. While we will also recommend yoga postures as part of healthy routines for children, care should be taken when introducing these exercises to children. We recommend first learning yoga postures with a certified teacher before taking up a practice on your own.

The information provided herein is for educational purposes based on traditional Ayurvedic practices and is not intended to prescribe, treat, diagnose, or provide medical advice for any treatment or disease. Always consult with a qualified physician for any medical problem.

PART ONE

Understanding Ayurveda

AN OVERVIEW

DEVELOPMENT OF MIND-BODY CONSCIOUSNESS IN CHILDREN

WHAT DOES IT mean to be a fully conscious parent—aware not only of your child's body, but of their mind *and* spirit? Many of you may have explored self-care through different wellness modalities like mindfulness, meditation, or yoga—perhaps also including Ayurveda—and you may have come to see the power of the mind-body-spirit connection in your own life and experienced firsthand the many benefits of embracing a more conscious lifestyle. Now that you're a parent seeking to extend that same awareness to your children and adopt wellness routines into your everyday parenting practices, you may be left looking for respected sources of information and ways to confidently implement these techniques to fully support the development of your children. Let's look at how to identify the mind-body connection in both you and your children.

Mind-Body Connection in Daily Life

Parenthood affords us many opportunities to consider the power of the mind-body health connection. Your children give you the gift of consistently bringing your attention back to the present moment from today's fast-paced world, allowing you to slow down and become mindful of the here and now. When this happens, you relax. Maybe you feel your shoulders soften, notice your breath slow and deepen, or even sense the tension in your facial muscles loosen. Suddenly you're smiling and feeling calm. Think about the time you spend putting your kids to bed. Speaking softly, reading a bedtime story, and simply slowing down in this evening routine may give you the feeling you have more to offer your children in those moments than you did all day. At times like these, it's easy to notice the tremendous influence your mind has over your physical body and how the positive effects of implementing mindfulness techniques to become present and calm the mind and body can improve the quality of your life and health.

Some days, it's easier to recognize the mind-body connection on the opposite extreme when it's triggered by stress. Even for parents who juggle childcare and after-school schedules with work and family life successfully most of the time, feelings of stress can creep in, leaving you overwhelmed and longing for more hours in the day to meet the demands of modern-day parenting. These feelings can derail your best efforts to maintain daily rhythms and a harmonious home or even lead to unhealthy changes in your sleep patterns, energy levels, or eating habits. With life sliding in and out of balance, it's easy to see the effects your mind and emotions have on your body and physical health.

Let's take a look at what happens. Maybe you had an interrupted night's sleep because you had to wake up multiple times and tend to a child, and the next day your patience wears thin when trying to finish a work assignment. Or a family member suddenly demands your attention, breaking your focus, and you feel your muscles seize or your heart race. This might cause you to lose your appetite or reach for something unhealthy to eat or lie awake worrying about the time you lost that day, setting yourself up for more fatigue. The interplay between mind and body is easy to recognize within yourself and obvious to you as examples of the mind-body connection. The same thing happens with your children—only they don't have the same awareness of it yet, and that's where you come in with Ayurvedic practices to support their developing mind-body system.

Ayurveda presents a body of knowledge on the role of this powerful connection for you to explore across different stages of your child's development and its influence on emotional health through thoughts and behaviors. This framework can help you cultivate a consistent, mindful approach to parenting that will promote vibrant and lasting health in your children.

Parenting Mindfully with Ayurveda

Striving to be a more conscious parent can sometimes seem a lofty ambition. Parenting more mindfully often means developing a keen awareness of the multitude of influencing factors that can impact your child's physical, emotional, and spiritual well-being on a daily basis. This can lead many parents to wonder how they can possibly find time to implement mindfulness techniques in their parenting practices without adding more stress to a life already at max capacity. Let's explore how.

Ayurveda provides parents a simple, multidimensional approach to balancing your child's body, mind, and spirit using natural and cost-effective practices. The application of Ayurveda in daily life is inviting and flexible and something every parent can bring into their home to establish and maintain wellness practices for the whole family. Throughout this book, we will explore daily routines, lifestyle tools, and everyday practices for your child, and later, discuss common childhood diseases and management of mind- and body-related disorders. One of the joys for parents discovering Ayurveda is that it never loses sight of the *whole child*—much like you—even while focusing on the separate components of body, mind, and soul.

AYURVEDA IN THE DIGITAL AGE

Parenting in the millennial age means perceiving and defining health differently than past generations and, for many individuals, expecting more from their health care. Many parents today are driven by a more proactive, preventive view of health and in search of a bridge between traditional and modern medicine that complements that perspective: something that closely resembles the multidimensional, individualized, and collaborative approach your child's doctor might take if he were both shaman and pediatrician. Perhaps that is how you came to read this book, searching out the best of both worlds, motivated by your own independent research online, reading books, and comparing notes with your circle of friends on the different resources available to help navigate your parenting journey. As you may have discovered, it's not always a simple path.

As parents can attest to better than anyone, life in the digital age often means being engulfed by information and feeling pulled in many directions at once. Simply researching a children's health remedy, for example, generates a stream of data and information from every corner of the globe—often causing more confusion. What starts out as a straightforward search query for a parenting tool can unwittingly turn into a never-ending quest to ensure your child's holistic development maps with the best advice every nation has to offer. This can compel parents to adopt more and more wellness routines in an effort to do the absolute best for their children, leading to even more uncertainty and not knowing where to turn. Maybe you've come to this through your own experience seeking natural healing remedies and alternatives, while longing to find the converging point for all these paths. The comprehensive science of Ayurveda helps parents both streamline and personalize their family's wellness plan as a complement to family health care, downsizing the information overload and setting children on a path to thrive. Let's look at how that works.

AYURVEDA AND YOUR CHILD

When exploring the role the mind-body connection plays in children's health, parents can wonder: With the impacts of the brain-body connection so profound in a fully grown adult, how are they affecting a developing child? And what will the effects be specifically on *my* developing child? Finally comes the million-dollar question—what can I do to promote positive development? A lot.

The collective knowledge and ancient wisdom of Ayurveda comprehensively answers these questions and forges a deeper understanding of the mind-body-spirit connection so you can live more consciously across all the aspects of your life. This offers you a gateway to create and maintain positive health, one family member at a time. In contrast to conventional medicine, Ayurveda assumes that we are actually *not* all identical on the inside or the outside and asserts the highest level of respect for each person's uniqueness. This belief strongly emphasizes that one size does not fit all when it comes to approaching health and well-being. In fact, it's quite the opposite.

Strikingly different from other systems of medicine, Ayurveda empowers the individual to know themselves and act from there. You are considered the healer, and Ayurveda, the science that supports you. This science is fully comprehensive and considers all aspects of a person's life—each no less important than the others. When creating individual wellness protocols, for example, Ayurveda takes a multidimensional view that reflects all the levels of an individual including the spiritual, physical, emotional, intellectual, behavioral, familial, environmental, and universal. Everyday health programs are then tailored around each of these components and to a person's unique body type and makeup—or prakriti—for a complete wellness plan.

This individualized approach to promoting health and managing disease offers parents the opportunity to apply the same fundamental techniques and guidelines to each of their children and simply fine-tune them according to each child's respective nature. Observing your children through this truly holistic lens encourages you to celebrate their uniqueness and true natures. It also invites you to view your whole child and the dynamic effects of the mind-body connection and how those may be manifesting across all of the different systems of your child's body.

One of the guiding principles at the helm of this holistic science—which we will explore shortly—is Ayurveda's health triad, which explains that mind, body, and soul are inseparable from their components, functioning together for better or worse—much like you and your children. When you view this triad as Ayurveda does—as inextricably connected from the very threshold of consciousness (before birth) and throughout a person's lifetime—you can clearly see the profound effects the mind-body-spirit relationship has on every stage of your child's development.

Ultimately, this framework offers you more ways to know your children and expands your parenting toolbox to include wisdom and strategies that may not have been passed down to you from earlier generations.

Ayurveda brings that generations-old wisdom into your home and gives you the comfort and confidence of having another support in place to meet your children's ever-shifting needs throughout every stage of childhood.

Ayurvedic Physiology

You may be wondering exactly how these influences can directly impact the functions of a child's body. This brings us to Ayurvedic physiology, a fascinating science that describes physiological function in terms of holistic health or a person's whole being. Whereas Western medicine primarily focuses on the structures of the physical body, Ayurveda centers around the energies *behind* the structures of the physical body and their ability to regulate and maintain each other in a *whole is greater than the sum of its parts* type of way. This synergy defines how these biophysical energy principles—or "functional energies" as they are termed—can enhance or diminish the functions of your child's body based on everyday experiences.

In this way, Ayurveda extends the reach of conventional Western medicine and offers a holistic perspective on physiological function to help you understand the ways you have more control over your child's health—and your own—than you might think. Once you have the context to better understand what is happening inside your child's body, this steers a more thorough examination of your lifestyle choices, some of which you may even currently regard as superficial. The more insight you gain from learning about the impacts and energetic reflections your child's environment and habits have on their various body systems, the more instinctive your choices will become.

Ayurveda's approach to health and physiology provides a stepping-stone to a higher state of wellness and integrates a system of proven science and ancient wisdom with modern medicine. It is important to note the two are perfectly compatible, and practicing one in no way excludes you from practicing the other. In fact, Ayurveda embraces the advances of modern science, working alongside Western medicine to provide individuals the most integrated, comprehensive care possible.

One of the greatest joys of adopting the principles of Kaumarabhritya, Ayurveda's branch of pediatrics, is the opportunity it provides parents to discover new dimensions to their children. For many parents, getting the green light to view and cultivate the physical health and mind of their child developing in sync opens up a great body of knowledge to reflect upon and emerge from with a pocketful of credible, holistic tools that can support your children's vitality and well-being.

Ayurveda's Health Triad: Body, Mind, Soul

The evolution of America's alternative and nonconventional medicine practices has catapulted quite a bit of ancient wisdom into mainstream health today. For many of you on a journey to embrace a more wellness-conscious lifestyle, it's no surprise to hear that you are not the body and you are not the mind, but instead a perfect union of body, mind, and soul.

For individuals and parents seeking a more balanced and natural way of living that promotes whole health, the concept of body, mind, and spirit being intimately entwined in a cosmic dance has become more familiar than extraordinary. In fact, you may already have an understanding of this paradigm from your own investigations into the mind-body connection as one continually suffused with impressions that will eventually materialize from consciousness into matter. In other words, all of your perceptions and inputs will at some point in time manifest physically or mentally in your mind or body. Perhaps that resonates with you on some level, but the nuances are hard to grasp. You may have simply settled for knowing the mind-body connection has the power to heal everything from your child's eczema to your own feelings of stress and anxiety—or sleeplessness, as one prominent example—and continued on with your wellness routines.

Ultimately, what you want to understand is how you can directly apply this knowledge of the mind-body connection in real time—across all the aspects of your daily life and the lives of your children. Exactly how does all this work morning, noon, and night? Enter Ayurveda.

As part science and part art of balanced daily living, what Ayurveda gives you—in addition to practical guidance—is routine and spirituality you can follow in your day-to-day life. The purpose of Ayurveda is to provide you the tools to achieve, maintain, and preserve health so you can live a long and happy life. Ayurveda emphasizes prevention of the imbalances that lead to disease as the most important way to achieve this goal and recognizes these imbalances can emanate from both the mind and the body. According to Ayurveda, prevention by definition is creating balance and functions as a science unto itself that sets forth guidelines and tools for resisting disharmony both internally and externally to maintain a state of health. Following Ayurvedic routines can help you establish rhythms in your child's daily life that align with these basic principles and connect us to nature to stay strong, harmonious, and balanced.

The first step on your journey toward whole family health is knowing that *you* are the primary healer. Ayurveda empowers everyone to take complete authority over their health and well-being. As a parent, you're operating from this threshold already—making Ayurveda your perfect counterpart. Once you learn a couple of foundational philosophies, what you will find is that these teachings, ancient as they may be, are actually quite intuitive. For example, now that you are familiar with the health triad, you understand that every individual is considered indivisible in mind, body, and spirit. When you view this oneness rising into existence from the moment of conception, you can see how your lifestyle patterns and choices have the ability to affect your child's development both inside and outside of the womb. Let's take a look at how it all begins.

THE BIRTH OF MIND, BODY, AND SPIRIT

Ayurveda views these three layers of the health triad as seamless and inseparable from conception, and their unbreakable union constitutes a human being. According to Ayurveda, human life begins at the single cell in the mother's womb that contains the entire *seed potential* to develop into a full-blown adult with a body, mind, and spirit. It's a concept you're already familiar with—how many times have you said yourself or heard someone say they can see the potential in someone or something? Just because it hasn't manifested yet doesn't mean it's not there. A whole tree is already there in the seed; it just hasn't emerged yet. It's the same with the seed potential of a cell—in this case, the zygote. The cell, just like the seed of a tree, simply needs to be nurtured and supported for a child to emerge. It is fascinating to recognize that the oneness of body, mind, and spirit is fixed from the moment of creation. Finally, when the conditions are optimal, the zygote is nurtured and a child is born. This is how Ayurveda comes to understands a child's body and mind as developing in tandem.

These layers of body, mind, and spirit support and hold each other together in a truly synergistic and magnetic way and cannot ever be separated—even if sometimes you'd like them to be—like when you lose your cool or someone hurts your child's feelings. The chain reaction across each of these layers of existence simply cannot be stopped. Comprehending the deep intelligence and mutual feeling integral to this paradigm helps parents understand that what underlies a child's state of health and well-being is the *harmony* of this triad. The key to unveiling your child's greatest potential—and the goal of healthy living—is preserving this balance. In the coming chapters we will explore different ways to identify and restore imbalances as they arise. First, though, let's look at why Ayurveda is so important in the lives of children.

Kaumarabhritya

Ayurveda's branch of pediatrics, Kaumarabhritya, explains early childhood as the most open, ready to nourish, ready to nurture stage of a human being's life. This is the period you can most effectively support every milestone of your children's development and, at the same time, help them to express their highest human potential throughout their lives.

What is the one thing in life you want most for your children? It is a universal truth that above all else, parents want their children to be healthy and happy and will do everything in their power to help them succeed. Often, it can be as simple as sharing your own happiness with them. How many times have you relayed a funny story to your child at the end of the day just to make them laugh and see them smile or shown them a picture of something that made you smile? It's instinctive to share the things that bring you joy with your children.

In the same way, it's instinctive to want to include your children in some of your daily wellness practices and lifestyle routines, like meditation or yoga—or even introduce them to various healing foods or herbs you may be exploring in your kitchen or garden. Perhaps you picked up this book to learn some new natural remedies and routines you could use at home or because of a growing concern you have over a particular condition affecting your child and are searching out additional resources. The teachings of Kaumarabhritya offer parents guidance on the prevention and management of various pediatric health conditions not based on physical symptoms alone, but according to the specific age and mind-body type of your child. You will learn how to identify your child's unique nature and determine their prakriti in the next chapter using a simple assessment chart and quiz that will serve as the basis of your Ayurvedic wellness protocols.

EARLY CHILDHOOD

The mind-body system in early childhood is like a sponge, absorbing every exposure as a direct download across all its receptors. What you may intuitively think happens is exactly what occurs: based on a multitude of exposures—which we will define in detail in coming chapters—and what is being absorbed, the mind-body system at some point starts reflecting these aspects back like a mirror. This is the way Ayurvedic science views our existence—as part of the cosmic existence. The human body is considered a mirror of our physical surroundings. In this way, everything external becomes internal. The everyday effects of different environments on your child's mind and body along with the inputs they receive in early childhood will influence their entire life. Their behavior, strengths, and even responses to stimuli like stress later in life will be based on how they were nurtured during the early childhood period.

Wouldn't it be nice if you could cherry-pick the best inputs of the day for your children to absorb? As a parent, it's difficult not to worry about the occurrences of incidents in your child's life that you may not have chosen and would remove if you could. As your children get older, or as you may already know if you have adolescents, spending more time away from home becomes the norm, and means you have even less control over what your child is exposed to day to day. Just as Ayurveda provides tools to optimize health, it also offers tools to minimize the negative effects of unwanted environmental or lifestyle exposures. Regardless of life's circumstances, there is much you can achieve using tailored, everyday Ayurvedic lifestyle tools to foster strength and vibrant health in your children, regardless of age.

Raising a child is a time in life when parents need a lot of support. There are so many aspects of their life to keep track of that it can sometimes be easy to lose sight of the big picture when managing the minutiae of issue after issue one at a time. The guidelines of Kaumarabhritya offer parents a way to effectively deal with the dynamic role of coordinating family health without ever inadvertently isolating any one part of your child. Take illness, for example. How many times have you treated your child's fever, then spent the rest of the day comforting them with your presence and providing them the emotional reassurances they needed to feel better? Physical remedies on their own are simply not enough. You can attest to this from your own experiences taking care of yourself as well. The nature and science of Ayurveda help you extend that same level of inner peace you feel when you know you are able to support your physical, mental, and spiritual needs to your children. It's bolstering to know they can benefit from this same harmony not only for their immediate growth and development but also for the future goal of transitioning to a healthy and happy adulthood.

Despite the day-to-day insanity that underlies raising young children—and the frequent, silent longings for a moment's peace in the bathroom—ultimately, there's nothing parents want more than to express their unconditional love to their children. Practicing Ayurveda with your children perfectly expresses that love and brings abundant joy and presence to your relationship. Ayurveda recognizes the "healthier your child, the happier they are" credo, making it the perfect companion for parents at every stage of childhood and, just as important, at every stage of parenthood.

AYURVEDA'S INVITATION TO PARENTS: COME AS YOU ARE

When parents first encounter natural healing systems like Ayurveda, they often feel guilty or even more stressed seeing all the ways they could have done better for their child. Becoming acquainted with the bright myriad of our mistakes is always humbling—and there is some burden that stems from all of this holistic learning!

It's natural to feel some anxiety when you come face-to-face with the profound influences the mind-body connection has on your child and the effects of certain lifestyle choices you may have made up to this point. However, one of the many things that makes Ayurveda so special is its perfect design to meet everyone who shows up exactly where they are; it is truly an open invitation to come as you are. If you have done the best you can for your child—which most parents are always doing based on the knowledge and awareness available to them at that point in time— there's no room for any regret or certainly any guilt. All that matters is what you're doing now, in the present moment. What you may come to find is that taking a more mindful approach to your parenting style will actually quiet a lot of self-doubt and bring with it a presence that is deeply connective and mutually nourishing for both you and your children. The guidelines and routines from the time-tested system of Ayurveda will not only be a comfort in the coming chapters but will also make you a more confident parent and your journey more fulfilling.

Assessing the Whole Child

What's the first thing your doctor assesses at a wellness visit? Is it your well-being? How about your mood or new tendencies and lifestyle patterns? Most likely they dive right into the physical symptoms assembly-line style to get you moving through the door where the remaining nine patients of the hour are waiting to be seen. If you're lucky, you will have established some modicum of personal connection with your doctor over the course of your relationship that doesn't leave you feeling in some way neglected or compelled to go home and begin searching online for more information. Modern-day medical appointments can sometimes feel both too clinical and too rushed.

Millions of parents today are embracing the use of natural remedies and complementary and alternative medicine (CAM) for the benefit of their children. The out-of-pocket spending alone of $1.9 billion a year on children ages four to seventeen—none of it covered by insurance—tells the story that conventional Western medicine is missing something. For many of today's health-conscious parents, holistic support for both mind and body, along with a patient-focused, collaborative health care experience, is not something they're willing to compromise on—especially when it comes to their children. Ayurveda fills in the gaps.

THE FABULOUS FOUR: COMPONENTS OF THE WHOLE CHILD

While modern health care systems essentially look at physical parameters to assess the health and development of an individual, Ayurveda explores the whole person—or whole child in this case—aligning with your own view of your children. These include the fabulous four: the physical, functional, mental, and emotional aspects of your child.

Let's look first at the physical, which we're all familiar with. Ayurveda considers the physical body as a carriage that supports the journey of the soul. Unique to Ayurveda is the interpretation of the term *body* to include both the physical and functional energies you just learned about in Ayurvedic physiology. The key is that Ayurveda assigns more importance to these functional aspects, whereas modern medicine focuses on the physical structures of the body alone.

According to Ayurveda, all of the functions of the physical body are carried out by functional energies—blood flowing through blood vessels, food transforming into nutrients, tissues forming from nutrients, etc. These energies are responsible for regulating all of the body's growth and development and even a person's vibrancy and energy levels. Think of these energies as the electricity that illuminates a bulb. Without that electrical energy, the bulb doesn't do anything. Similarly, an organ without functional energies does not fulfill its functions in the physical body.

Let's take a look at how this works. The cells and tissues in our structural body are constantly degenerating due to wear and tear and completion of their life cycles while at the same time being newly constructed through cellular nutrition. One hundred twenty days is the optimal life of a red blood cell in the body. Childhood, however, is a different story because this is a period when the building of new tissue needs to be carried out faster than the wear and tear and other degenerative processes naturally occurring in the body. In this stage of life, the required ratio of tissue building over degeneration is not the same as for adults, and a greater skew toward building is essential for the optimal development of various organ systems and growth of a child. This is where functional energies come in. When one of the functional energies becomes imbalanced—due to lifestyle or environment, let's say—it can compromise the function of one or more of the body's systems and affect a child's development.

In the same way you have come to understand the oneness of body and mind, you can also grasp the relationship between the physical body and functional energies: they are similarly intertwined and supportive of each other. Every physical structure of the body is designed to accomplish a function, and at the same time, every healthy structure is the outcome of a functional process. In other words, healthy function is what maintains an organ or body system. When the functions of the body are negatively affected, it can result in the structural alteration of that organ or system. For example, increased blood pressure often causes enlargement of the heart chambers or damage to the kidney cells. The goal of Ayurveda is to keep the energies responsible for the functions of the physical body in balance.

Understanding these energies at work in your child on a physical, functional, mental, and emotional level can help you support them throughout this all-important age of development. Ayurveda explains that body and mind are always working together as a single unit, and any ripple in the mind influences the body and vice versa. Because of this, assessing and understanding a child's mental and emotional status helps in the personalization of guidance based on the unique nature and needs of the child.

The Three Functional Energies

What makes a clock tick or a bulb illuminate? We obviously know it's not the clock or the bulb itself. In the same way, you can understand that the basis of Ayurvedic physiology rests on the functional energies behind the physical body—and not *with* the physical body. Knowing these energies govern all of the body systems and can enhance or diminish function according to their state of equilibrium can help you see just how much influence you have over your child's health.

On its own, modern medicine leaves the impression that beyond basics like staying hydrated or taking a daily regimen of supplements (more on that later), individuals have almost no control over the physiological systems and functions of their bodies. This perception alone can create feelings of vulnerability and helplessness that often exacerbate any health conditions you might be dealing with or that may arise. This can be especially defeating for parents facing an illness or disorder of any magnitude impacting their child. Discovering the ways functional energies can influence specific physiologic processes of the body along with the different ways you can help keep them in balance offers you many ways to support your children's health and well-being.

Ayurveda invites you to discover the definition of health and immunity from a new framework. According to the Vedic texts, health expands far beyond the absence of illness and infirmity and is best be looked at from the perspective of living a fulfilling and blissful life.

Ayurveda defines health as the balanced state of the functional principles (*dosha*), digestion and metabolism (*agni*), optimally nourished tissues (*dhatu*), and elimination (*malakriya*) with a pleasant and vibrant soul, the senses, and the mind. This harmony on the inside helps resist disharmony on the outside to prevent disease—Ayurveda's definition of immunity. There are three types of functional energies that govern all of the functions of the body, and it is their balanced union that maintains health. On the flip side, any imbalance in these functional energies—whether excess or deficiency—can lead to a state of disease, thereby causing qualitative changes in physiological functions. You may already be somewhat familiar with these doshas, as the term has become popular in wellness circles. Let's look at them a little more closely.

THE DOSHAS

The energy that governs the age of childhood is *kapha*, the glue energy that holds everything together. This energy principle supports the integrity of tissues, nourishment, and stability of a child. A deficiency of kapha leads to lack of nourishment or thinness, whereas an excess can cause weight gain and congestion. The second energy principle is *pitta,* the fire energy that cooks. Pitta facilitates transformation, digestion, metabolism, and warmth. The depletion of pitta can slow down digestion and metabolism, causing lethargy, whereas too much pitta can lead to excessive heat in the body that expresses as anger or a fever, for example. The master principle energy responsible for all flow, movement, and activity is *vata,* the energy of vibration. A deficiency of vata can slow down flow, enthusiasm, and activity, whereas the excess may lead to restlessness, dryness, and inconsistencies in body functions.

As we continue to explore the doshas in the following chapters, you will become familiar with the specific ways these shifting energies can affect your child's entire system and the importance of keeping them in harmony. While the doshas each have their own independent qualities that continually influence the mind-body system, they also work together as a group to carry out different functions of the body's various systems.

Sometimes they work in pairs, and at others all three operate together—either supporting the key principle of one dosha or a single body function as a group. For example, vata dosha governs the principle of movement and is independently responsible for the functions of inhalation, exhalation, and the exchange of oxygen and carbon dioxide in the respiratory system. In this case, kapha supports vata by providing the moistness and mucous lining essential for the smooth functioning of breathing. In the case of digestion, the doshas work all together: Vata transports all of the body's digestive secretions to the stomach and carries out movement of the gut. Pitta facilitates the production of digestive acids and transformation of food into nutrients. And kapha provides the protective lining of the stomach, which holds everything in its proper place.

You might be wondering how you can possibly keep all of these energies in balance all of the time. First, Ayurveda gives you a viewfinder of sorts to bring the doshas clearly into focus. Once these energies become visible, you can then assess the state of your child's doshas and choose from many different techniques to restore balance as needed by integrating the natural principles of Ayurvedic diet, lifestyle, and routine we will discuss. Over time, you will find that balancing the doshas will become quite intuitive. Often it's as simple as listening to your body—like putting on a sweater if you're chilly, for example, or making a trip to the bathroom when you first feel the urge to eliminate.

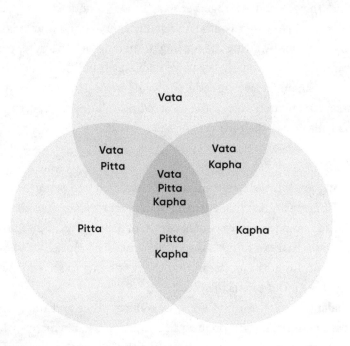

The doshas are not only present inside us, but in everything around us, and this reveals the many ways Ayurveda connects us to nature. In the next chapter, we will continue to explore the effects of the doshas on the different cycles and rhythms of life. This will help you create daily and seasonal routines for your family that harmonize with the natural cycles of these energies.

Your Child's Mind and Body Are One

The next time your child walks in the room, try and picture their mind and body strolling toward you hand in hand. Ayurveda views your child much like you do—whole, not separated in mind or body.

Now picture your child having a temper tantrum or some other form of emotional meltdown. Does the saying "out of one's mind" sound fitting? In those moments, this is literally true for your child. They are not present, and both mind and body are on another planet, so to speak—but they are still together, illustrating again how they cannot be separated. Just as they leave together, they come back together. Maybe you've noticed this yourself in the moments following an outburst. As you begin to bring your child's body back into balance by giving them a hug or rubbing their back, for example, the mind follows. Similarly, when you start to bring the mind back into balance by singing a favorite song or playing some gentle music, the body follows. Your children express the tremendous role and influence the mind and body have over their lives moment to moment.

YOUR CHILD'S MIND

According to Ayurveda, the mind is considered the sense beyond the senses. This means it is the sense that *first* perceives happiness or sadness; feelings of being relaxed or restless, content or longing; and so on. When you consider that the mind is responsible for all of your child's emotions and perceptions of the world around them, it's easy to see why Ayurveda teaches that "mind care is life care."

A balanced state of mind not only reflects peace and tranquility but also leads your child to respond to all stimuli in a stable manner. In turn, this supports proper function across all of the systems of the body. A balanced mind has the ability to focus, perceive, and register information gathered and also to retain and recollect that information when associated within context. It is important to note that when it comes to learning, every child has a different level of ability—for both retaining and processing. This simply makes them unique. The modern world's one standard for all approach to learning construes these diversified abilities as deficiencies or problems. However, supporting every child's unique approach and ability to learn fuels their esteem, and that is when they perform much beyond expectations.

Conversely, when your child's mind is out of balance, almost anything happening around them can bring on negative emotions. How many times have you seen your child morph into a monster and respond with anger, frustration, or jealousy to seemingly nothing in a totally unexpected way? We often watch our children behave in strange ways when they are emotionally affected by something—not showing their usual interests when returning home from school, turning down their favorite meals, and other outputs of that nature. Those can all be taken as signs that the mind is out of balance. We will explore the different ways you can take care of your child's five senses to support clear perception and a balanced mind later in the book.

MIND-BODY INFLUENCE

As hard as it is to imagine the countless times a day this happens, the mind and body influence each other each and every time they encounter various stimuli. *Every time.* Understanding how changes in the physical body influence the mind and how emotional influences impact the physical body is key to maintaining your child's health. For instance, a child showing no interest in eating their favorite meal or getting easily frustrated over something small will most likely express physically that same day with constipation or some other ailment. Think about the effects on your child's mind and behavior when they get hurt and sustain a physical injury, after excessive exertion, or even when the weather changes or they feel hungry. These common expressions unquestionably confirm the unceasing influences of mind and body.

Dr. J has seen many children in his practice with chronic eczema, for example, who express increased irritability and moodiness and have frequent tantrums. The way they respond even during a consultation reflects the effects of their skin irritation on their mind. There is simply no separating conditions of the mind and body; they are one and the same.

Another common example of children expressing imbalances pivots around nutrition. Parents often come to Dr. J with nutritional concerns: either their children aren't eating enough, or despite eating plenty, they may still be underweight or show other signs of poor growth. We will explore this subject in depth in part two of this book, but for now you can understand this as an expression of disharmony or imbalance in the functional energies. Even though you may give your child an adequate quantity of food that represents an ideal ratio of nutrients and calories, that doesn't guarantee proper digestion and absorption. And—most surprising to some—neither do high-quality organic ingredients. What is essential then for a child's nourishment? Mind care. The quality of care and time you spend with your child and the patience you show them along the way with your supportive and encouraging responses play a role equal to food when it comes to nutrition.

Considering the mutual influence of the body and mind gives parents an essential framework for understanding their children and allows them to approach their health and well-being in a comprehensive way, even at times when the connection is not so obvious. For example, you may not think your ability to avoid conflicts with your children and with others in front of them matters outside of protecting their emotional health and vibrancy, but the reality is this also supports their balanced digestion and nourishment. That, in turn, will not only support the physical strength they need but also the mental strength—and both contribute to a healthy immune system that will help them sustain high stressors in their life to come.

The core strength of a child's whole life is developed through proper management of the mind-body system in childhood. While Ayurveda clearly sets forth and defines a multitude of tools available to support the balanced development of a child including diet, lifestyle, herbs, and natural remedies that we will explore in detail throughout this book, it is essential to remember that if you are focused on body only, or mind only, a complete state of health cannot be attained.

As we move on now to explore the doshas and identify your child's constitution, remember that Ayurveda is not a prescription, rather it is designed to reveal how important it is to enjoy life and remind you of all the ways you are already in the flow of nature. Dr. J can assure you based on years of experience guiding parents that simply sharing these insights with your children and spending time relaxing and enjoying life's moments with them will naturally bring you both the best life has to offer.

2

UNDERSTANDING YOUR
CHILD'S TRUE NATURE

THERE'S NOTHING PARENTS pride themselves on more than knowing their children better than anyone—on occasion even better than they know themselves! How many times have you instinctively understood what's best for your children based on your vast catalog of impressions and unmatched experiences with them? Your insights as a parent are powerful and allow you a kaleidoscopic view of who your children truly are moment to moment as the world turns around them and their environments shift. These luminous reflections reveal every dimension of what makes your children so innately special and give you countless insights into their true nature. Tuning in to these expressions with close attention is accepting the invitation to the unequaled journey of parenting with mindfulness and is a true gift to your children, just as they are a gift to you.

Parents instinctively note their children's innermost strengths, talents, desires, and vulnerabilities, as well as remarkable differences between siblings from a very early age. In fact, the contrasts between children born in the same family is downright fascinating. Even a quick study can leave a parent wondering how one toddler can play happily on the beach all day in the hot sun while another quickly becomes red-faced and irritable. Much like two different seeds planted in the same soil, everything born on this earth carries its own specific true nature. You see this everywhere you go.

Your awareness of your children's tendencies, characteristics, and dominant traits will allow you to discover your child's true nature—the fundamental key to understanding and maintaining positive health and well-being according to Ayurveda. Not only will this give you the opportunity to implement wellness protocols according to your child's unique constitution, it will help strengthen the connection between you and your children—something every parent strives for on each leg of the parenting journey. Let's take a look through the Ayurvedic lens and learn how you can unlock your child's potential.

Ayurveda's most important tool for formulating daily lifestyle routines along with prevention and treatment plans is recognizing the inborn nature of a child. This fundamental principle invites you to heighten your awareness of the present moment and adopt parenting strategies at various stages of your children's development that best complement and suit their inborn constitution. As you probably know from your own experience, medicine isn't one-size-fits-all, and in the same way, there isn't one way to parent any two children. On top of that, what works today won't necessarily work tomorrow! Staying present while tuning in to your child's unique mind-body expressions will not only bring you closer, but will also support you to be more proactive, flexible, and prepared for the multitude of situations that arise in your busy, often unpredictable life as a parent.

Prakriti

Ayurveda recognizes a person's true nature as their *prakriti*, or constitution—the inseparable aspect of existence and unique nature of an individual. This constitution is established at the time of conception and remains the same throughout a person's lifetime regardless of any impacts that arise from health or lifestyle. You might be wondering if your own constitution determines your child's constitution, but prakriti arises on its own. Even if both parents have a vata constitution, as an example, it does not necessarily follow that their child will be vata-predominant. Prakriti does not indicate an imbalance or anything that needs fixing and will not cause any disease on its own. It is, instead, a blueprint for understanding your child's bodily structures and functions along with their tendencies and affinities.

Why is it necessary to understand your child's prakriti? Isn't it enough that you know your child needs white noise and a certain stuffy to sleep, or the crust cut off their sandwich at lunchtime, or the tub filled with an exact ratio of bubbles to water if you want them to get in without a struggle? Yes and no. Every grain of knowledge and perception you have absorbed since the day your child was born will contribute to understanding their unique constitution, but there is more to explore. Knowing your children's prakriti can pinpoint propensities for specific illnesses and disorders, for example. Tuning in every day to your child's various expressions will cue you to any current imbalances, known as *vikriti*, that may be present and can even help prevent disease in early stages—in many cases, long before trouble arises. This essential Ayurvedic tool is your guide to recognizing and balancing the subtle channels of your child's mind-body system so you can adapt to their constantly shifting needs.

Ayurveda discusses prakriti in terms of the three doshas we just learned about as the functional energies behind the physical body: vata, pitta, and kapha. The structural and functional nature of your child's body systems along with their tendencies and affinities will vary to a great extent according to this prevailing energy. This is why understanding your child's unique constitution is essential for determining Ayurvedic daily routines. Simply put, what is healthy for one child may not be healthy for another, even if they're siblings. Let's begin with a snapshot of the doshas.

If a child is born with a vata-predominant constitution, their nature will express more vata-related qualities and tendencies. These children can seem very active and comparatively restless to other constitutions because vata governs the principle of movement. It can be hard to sit still and relax when your mind-body system is always in a state of vibration. In the same way, you may notice expressions of heat and sharpness in children governed by pitta, the principle of fire and transformation. Out of balance, these children are prone to anger and jealousy, for example. Finally, kapha-dominant constitutions often exhibit marked calmness and endurance due to the governing energy of cohesion and binding. A kapha child often appears content and more patient than other children but, out of balance, may exhibit signs of laziness.

Ayurveda's definition of health fundamentally rests on maintaining the unique and innate combination of the doshas you were born with. In other words, balance doesn't mean striving for equal parts vata, pitta, and kapha, but rather *sustaining* the ratio your child was born with. Please keep in mind that one dosha is not better than the other and, in balance, every individual will express their highest vibration of potential across mind, body, and spirit.

As you learn to recognize different doshic expressions across your child's mind-body system and study the Ayurvedic Constitution Charts on the following pages, you'll be amazed to see how profound your insights as a parent have been all along! Chances are, you will discover that following your instinctive beliefs and solutions for how to best raise your children likely prove to be part of a parenting paradigm that perfectly aligns with your child's constitution. After all, you know them best.

It is important to note that it is not necessary for your child to express all of the characteristics of a particular dosha. Dominant doshas are identified by recognizing predominant characteristics and qualities attributed to a specific constitution type and will be obvious to you as a parent. Once you spot this combination, you will be ready and able to adapt a multitude of simple strategies that can help you support optimal health using your child's true nature as your guide.

Vata: The One That Governs Movement

The chart below summarizes the most common characteristics of vata dosha, along with aggravating factors, disorder tendencies, and principles of management.

Characteristics	Vata children are generally slim and slender and comparatively more difficult to nourish and build tissues; either short or tall with prominent joints.
	General physical characteristics are oval face, small eyes, dry skin, thin hair, small joints (may crack often), and long fingers.
	Variability is vata's nature; their metabolism and sleep patterns are always changing.
	They talk a lot, move a lot, and are generally restless most of the time; they use lots of hand gestures.
	They attract other children with their talkative and expressive nature.
	They are very intuitive, imaginative, and artistic. They enjoy writing poems, creating art, and dancing.
	They are always on the go and love to travel.
	The vata mind is like a busy bee, constantly buzzing around, moving in circles. They are born worriers and often worry about anything and everything.
	They often feel anxious and nervous. Many times, their mind is in the future, not enjoying the present moment.
Causes of Aggravation	Cold and dry weather; prone to aggravation in the fall season and early part of winter
	Eating too many dry, bitter, pungent, astringent, light, or processed foods
	Consuming cold food and beverages
	Exposure to cold and wind
	Listening to loud noise, bright lights, excessive TV or computer use
	Erratic sleep schedules
	Fasting, irregular dieting; insufficient or interrupted sleep
	Staying up late; holding on to natural urges such as the urge to urinate or empty bowels
	Stress, fear, anxiety, insecurity, worry

Disorder Tendencies	Dryness of skin, hair, eyes, ears, lips, stools; bloating and gas; dehydration
	Restless mind, flightiness; dizziness, thinness, tendency to be underweight
	Cold body, poor circulation, muscle cramps, constriction, tightness, pain, asthma
	Cracking of skin and lips
	Irregular movements, shivering, muscle twitching, fear, anxiety, insecurity
	Restlessness, fast actions, chatter, fidgeting
	Racing and agitated mind
Principles of Management	Favor sweet, sour, and salty tastes.
	Avoid cold food and beverages, minimize leftovers, and enjoy warm, moist meals.
	Ensure optimal hydration by drinking warm water, broths, and soups.
	Incorporate rich, healthy fats into diet such as olive oil, avocado oil, sesame oil, and clarified butter.
	Apply natural moisturizers and heavy oils to the body 20 minutes before bathing or after thoroughly dry from shower.
	Avoid overexertion from exercise; engage in relaxing board games and low-intensity activities.
	Go to bed early and avoid late nights.

Pitta: The One That Produces Heat

The chart below summarizes the most common characteristics of pitta dosha, along with aggravating factors, disorder tendencies, and principles of management.

Characteristics	Pitta children have a medium build with strong tissues.
	Sharpness is a main characteristic—sharp nose, sharp eyes, sharp chin, and sharp tongue.
	Pitta children are often good speakers; concise and direct.
	They are precise, goal-oriented, orderly, and tidy.
	Pitta children are list makers, do everything based on a plan, are always punctual.
	The pitta mind is like a bull. Once it is made up, it is difficult to change.
	They are often opinionated, criticizing others, telling children what is right and wrong.
	Pittas get irritable or angry quickly, especially when things do not go their way.
	Metabolism is very sharp; as the saying goes, they are always hungry or angry!
Causes of Aggravation	Hot weather
	Eating too many sour, salty, or pungent foods; too much yogurt, sour juices, junk food
	Too much sun and heat
	Anger, irritability, and frustration
	Excessive competition, intellectual stimulation
Disorder Tendencies	Nausea, vomiting, diarrhea, oily skin, acne, skin blisters
	Gastritis, acidity, heartburn
	Irritability, anger, sharp headaches
	Fevers, infections, inflammations; red, hot eyes
	Sensory sensitivity to heat and light, ringing in ears
	Strong acidic odor to feces, sweat and urine, skin, breath
	Excessive perspiration and thirst

Principles of Management	Favor sweet, astringent, and bitter tastes and minimize sour items including vinegars, yogurt, and salty, hot, and spicy foods.
	Eat more fresh fruit and cooling vegetables such as squash and leafy greens and minimize acidic fruits such as sour oranges.
	Ensure optimal hydration through drinking fresh juices, milk, buttermilk, and water at room temperature.
	Avoid excessive exposure to sun and heat and try to relax and engage in indoor activities on hot summer days.

Kapha: The One That Adheres and Builds

The chart below summarizes the most common characteristics of kapha dosha, along with aggravating factors, disorder tendencies, and principles of management.

Characteristics	Kapha children are well built and sometimes overweight.
	Physical features are rounded—round face, big, round eyes, roundish nose, and sweet looks; long, thick hair.
	Kapha children are loving, nurturing, and caring.
	They are peacemakers; they want everybody to be happy.
	They have strong endurance and immune systems.
	They are good listeners and speak little; tend to be shy at times.
	A bit lazy, kapha-type personalities like to rely on and follow others.
	They have slow minds; often focused in the past.
	Kapha children get easily attached and have a hard time letting go.
Causes of Aggravation	Cold and wet weather; late winter, spring, and the rainy season
	Eating too many sweet, sour, or salty foods
	Junk food such as candy, ice cream, desserts, doughnuts, oily/fried foods, red meat, excessive milk, and cheese products
	Excessive eating and drinking
	Excessive sleep
	Lack of exercise or physical activity
Disorder Tendencies	Clammy skin
	Cold body; colds, cough, congestion
	Heaviness, obesity
	Slow digestion
	Laziness, excessive sleep, lethargy
	Excessive saliva in the mouth, white-coated tongue
	Water retention
	Comparatively slow thinking

Principles of Management	Increase pungent, astringent, and bitter tastes.
	Include warm foods and beverages; avoid cold foods and beverages.
	Eat more baked, cooked, or grilled food and minimize oily and fried items.
	Incorporate healthy spices including turmeric, ginger, and garlic known to enhance digestion, metabolism, and circulation.
	Stay physically active as part of a daily regimen and minimize sedentary activities and games.
	Avoid or minimize daytime sleep.

How the Doshas Connect Your Child to Nature

One of the best ways to learn how to see the doshas clearly in your children—as well as yourself—is to begin to recognize them in the world around you. Ayurveda considers all living beings to be one with nature, providing the perfect lens for observing the unique qualities and characteristics of the doshas at work in the universe. Let's take a look at this framework so you can begin to bring your child's doshas into focus.

Have you ever characterized your child as restless as the wind or as fiery as the sun? Ayurveda recognizes the human body as a mirror not only of our physical surroundings in elemental composition, but also of the same dynamic energies of the three doshas expressed in the cosmos. As you discover the different ways the doshas manifest in your environment and surroundings, you will begin to notice the impact of their influences and rhythms on your child's mind and body.

From sunrise to sunset, to daily rhythms and changing seasons—and even the stages of life itself—these continually shifting energies and their impacts remind us that the only constant in life is change. Daytime, for example, brings the heating and stimulating energy of the sun, which creates warmth and raises our body temperature, whereas nighttime carries the cooling and soothing energy of the moon that helps us to feel relaxed and grounded. Similarly, you can identify different qualities of the doshas according to season. Summer represents heat, while springtime produces wetness, and fall and winter are marked by dryness and cold. These constantly shifting exposures in our environment influence the interplay and equilibrium of the doshas within our own bodies, challenging us to maintain balance.

This brings us to the very definition of *dosha*—literally "that which can go out of balance." This is the key concept of all three doshas and the foundation of your Ayurvedic tool kit. Once you learn to identify these specific energies and keep an eye on their influences, you can adjust your children's daily and seasonal regimens and lifestyle routines to maintain equilibrium according to their unique constitutions. In harmony, the doshas create a state of perfect health; out of balance, they can cause disorder and disease.

You may be wondering at this point how you can possibly keep your child's energies balanced when there are so many influences out of your control. Ayurveda provides simple strategies for both stabilizing and neutralizing the external impacts of the world around you and emphasizes prevention as a way to generate balance all on its own. Let's take a deeper look now at the expressions and qualities of the three doshas and different ways you can adapt to their rhythms.

DANCING WITH THE DOSHAS

Ayurveda identifies a key principle that can help you stay in step with the doshas and prevent possible imbalances: *Like increases like and opposites create balance.* Let's take a look next at some examples illustrating this principle at work.

A hot summer day, for example, increases pitta—the energy of fire and transformation. Sending your child outside to play a game of soccer in the midday sun will increase the heat within their body. This isn't necessarily a bad thing—but depending on your child's constitution, it could result in an accumulation of excess pitta, especially if that is your child's constitution. Drinking a cool beverage and sitting in the shade will pacify pitta, whereas sunbathing will aggravate it and make it harder to restore balance. Similarly, shuttling your child to and from multiple activities every day after school increases vata—the energy of movement. If vata is your child's dominant dosha, this can lead to an imbalance, particularly in the windy and dry fall season. Drinking a cold breakfast smoothie will further aggravate vata, whereas drinking a cup of warm tea will help to pacify the dosha. A kapha child suffers from excess cold and wetness. A winter's night meal served with ice water followed by a bowl of ice cream for dessert, for instance, will increase the qualities of kapha and produce an imbalance depending on constitution type. Remember, like increases like and opposites create balance!

Once you tune in to the frequency of the doshas, you will begin to see them everywhere, and many of Ayurveda's tools and techniques for restoring balance will come quite naturally. The power of Ayurveda unfolds exactly this way—perfectly aligning you with nature and escorting you into the present moment where you are rewarded with the joys of mindfulness, the greatest gift you can give to your children.

THE FIVE ELEMENTS

Now that you understand prakriti as the inseparable, true nature of an individual and the three doshas at work governing all the systems and functions of your child's body, you may be wondering about the physical structures of your child's body. What do the doshas have to do with healthy bone and muscle growth, tissue development, joint integrity, brain health, gut health, and overall neurological development?

This brings us to the concept of the five elements. Ayurveda explains that everything in the cosmos is constructed by five fundamental elements: Earth, Water, Fire, Air, and Space. These elements are considered the fundamental building blocks or construction units of everything in nature and the universe—including our physical bodies. In other words, the same materials exist both within us and outside us on this earth. This is the fundamental reason for the seamless expression of nature's influences on your child's mind, body, and spirit. Let's take a brief look at how the doshas and the five elements are connected.

When you consider the five elements—beyond the substance and matter, Ayurveda recognizes that each of them carries unique energies or qualities, just like the doshas. In fact, those qualities give rise to the three doshas. Earth and Water, for example, have qualities of being heavy and stable, or binding and building. This may sound familiar to you from what you've learned about kapha. That is because kapha is composed of Earth and Water. What about pitta—the principle of heat and transformation? Pitta is composed of the Fire and Water elements. You might be wondering how that makes sense when water extinguishes fire? An open fire is rampant and uncontrollable. Left alone, it will burn and devastate everything in its path. The Water element of pitta helps contain the Fire element so that it is still active but sustainable. Last, vata—the principle of movement—is derived from the subtlest elements: Air and Space. This is why dry and windy weather aggravates vata—because of the increase in mobile, fast-moving qualities.

CONNECTING THE DOTS

As you can see, the doshas are the functional expression of the five elements that provide a framework for understanding the structural makeup of existence. In the same way structure and function are interdependent, so are anatomy and physiology. A balanced vata dosha supports the normal function of every physiological process within your child's body that is governed by vata and requires movement—both voluntary and involuntary. This includes physical movement, peristaltic movement of the digestive tract, muscle contractions, and even the movement of thoughts. In the same way, a balanced pitta dosha sustains normal digestion, metabolism, hormonal changes, body temperature, and energy levels. Kapha in balance supports the integrity and cohesion of all the organ systems and tissues of the body along with proper nourishment.

When you picture the doshas circulating within your body, you can note the fascinating interdependence of structure and function. Proper production of digestive enzymes, for example, ensures the nourishment of tissue, bone, and muscle. It is important to note here that when a normal function within the body is hindered in some way by doshic imbalances, structural changes can occur over time.

The more closely you observe the doshas in your child's day-to-day mind and body expressions, the better you will be able to support their health and vitality. After just a short time, it will become instinctive. Your senses will sharpen as you tune in to the rhythms of nature, and this awareness will guide you day by day throughout your parenting journey.

Before you take the quiz at the end of this chapter to discover your child's prakriti, I want to highlight the various cycles of the doshas in the world around us. This will help you develop a clear picture of nature's influences on your child, identify potential causes of imbalance, and adapt lifestyle choices according to the flow of nature. Why swim against the current when you can ride the tide? Parenting bears enough challenges on its own. Ayurveda makes it easier.

o o o

Ayurvedic Root Principle: Like Increases Like

Same qualities always cause increase, and opposite qualities, reduction. Adding heat to warm water makes it hotter, whereas adding cold reduces the warmth.

o o o

Doshas and the Seasons

How many times have you bundled your child up on a fall morning before school only to have them come home at the end of the day growling at you as they race to change into a pair of shorts? Who knew that chilly fall morning would turn into a beach day? No wonder your kid is mad! Anger is an expression of aggravated pitta.

The seasonal cycle of the doshas gives you a three-dimensional blueprint for recognizing various influences of nature on your child's mind-body system. When you look out your window through an Ayurvedic lens, you can quite literally see that what is happening on the outside is also happening on the inside. In the same way daily routines can help establish proper rhythms in your child's life, Ayurveda recommends following seasonal routines throughout the year. This will help you attune your child's lifestyle practices to each season's doshic qualities and give you another tool to keep the doshas in balance. External influences can affect everything from your child's immunity to their overall disposition.

Let's begin with summertime. The rising heat impacts the human body just as it does the earth. As this heat accumulates in the body, it increases the probability of heat-related health issues and disorders including acidity, skin inflammation, and even blazing tempers. You can easily observe the *like increases like* principle at work here and spot how pitta can quickly become aggravated this time of year. When fall arrives with windy, dry, and colder weather, the increase in mobile qualities can aggravate vata in the same way. A vata imbalance commonly manifests across the mind-body system as dry skin, digestive irregularities, mental restlessness, and increased aches and pains. Do you ever feel like hibernating in the winter and sitting on your couch until spring? The cold, frozen, and static qualities of wintertime can increase kapha and create sluggishness or heaviness in the body. Our system shields itself to preserve internal heat and ward off the impacts of the cold weather. This enhances digestion and explains why there is a tendency to eat more during the winter. When the frozen ground and ice begin to melt in springtime, wetness spreads across nature much the same way it spreads throughout our bodies in the forms of congestion and accumulation. Metabolism slows and dampens. This process can weaken the immune system, leaving your child prone to springtime allergies.

Remember, when it comes to modifying lifestyle routines according to season, it is best to step outside and tune in to nature rather than relying on the calendar!

Doshas and Daily Time Cycles

Do you have a child who tends to wake up congested early in the morning or has trouble getting out of bed for school? The same way the seasons create different energies both within and around us, so do the dynamics of the sun, the moon, and the earth. As you can see from the illustration on p. 44, you can recognize these different qualities in the daily cycle of the doshas over a twenty-four-hour period.

Early morning, for example, is considered a kapha time. Your child is more likely to feel sluggish or heavy between these hours and may have an especially hard time waking up—especially if they are kapha-predominant. As the sun comes out and rises higher in the sky, feelings of dullness and heaviness decrease as the warmth of the sun takes over. This heat enhances the entire mind-body system and increases clarity, activity, and the digestive fire—just in time for lunch. Pitta peaks at noon and is the ideal time to have a heavy meal as digestion is at its strongest. As the sun goes down and the heat of the day diminishes, vata moves in with colder temperatures and qualities of dryness, representing the period of late afternoon.

Do you have a tendency to wake up in the middle of the night tossing and turning? The same way daytime begins with kapha in the morning, peaks with pitta, and ends with vata, this same cycle occurs at night. Kapha dominates the evening, pitta peaks at midnight, then vata takes over until early morning. Did you know vata governs elimination? This explains patterns of insomnia or a consistent need to use the bathroom

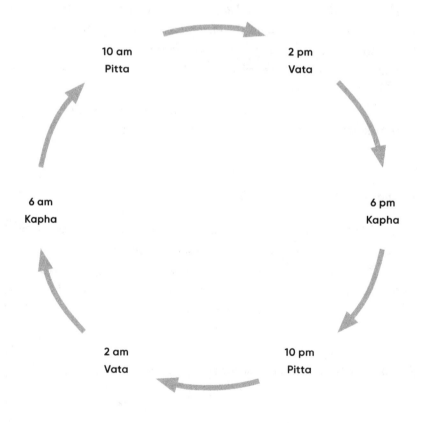

10 am
Pitta

2 pm
Vata

6 am
Kapha

6 pm
Kapha

2 am
Vata

10 pm
Pitta

during these hours. Expressions like these can cue you in to potential imbalances.

Following the cycle of the doshas in four-hour increments throughout the day allows you to understand their effects on your child's mind-body system based on time of day. Children who are highly emotional, for example, may be a little more sensitive when the clock strikes noon. Similarly, children with a tendency toward restlessness should be soothed with a warming beverage or cuddle in the late afternoon. These types of routines can pacify imbalances that may be accumulating. Prevention is key.

Doshas and the Cycle of Life

Finally, we come to the cycle of life itself. Even this corresponds to the rise and fall of the doshas. Ayurvedic science explains that kapha dominates childhood; pitta, the stage of midlife; and vata, the period of old age.

During childhood, the overarching influence of kapha governs children regardless of their constitution. This is important for parents to recognize so that you can help prevent imbalances associated with this stage of life and understand why it is vital your children are well-nourished on every level to support this period of rapid growth and development. Do you feel like you're always at the doctor with one of your kids for a sinus or ear infection? Disorder tendencies during this time of life include congestion, excess mucus, coughs, and frequent colds. You may notice your child suffers more from these illnesses than their vata and pitta counterparts if they have a kapha-predominant constitution. You probably recognize by now how the accumulation of the cold, damp qualities of kapha increases in the winter, heightening the likelihood children could develop associated illnesses. We will look more closely at the influences of kapha dosha on children in the next chapter.

The pitta dosha represents the next stage of life—the transformational period of early adulthood. This time is dominated by the fire energy and qualities of high intensity, motivation, determination, drive, and courage. There's no question these attributes predominate this stage of life and, in fact, make it possible to strike out on your own, establish a career, and start a family. Finally, vata dominates the period of old age associated with depletion and dryness you can easily associate with degenerative changes and painful disorders of the mind and body, a reflection of accumulated dryness and increased vata.

Now that you are familiar with the dynamic role of the doshas and their unique characteristics, it's time for you to identify your child's prakriti—the key to implementing all of the Ayurvedic tools and techniques you will discover throughout this book.

Child's Prakriti Quiz

The following quiz will help you identify your child's Ayurvedic constitution. Please remember this assessment should not be used to diagnose any health problems your child may have; rather, it is a way to better understand your child's overall nature and guide you to create customized lifestyle routines using various Ayurvedic tools and techniques.

Answer the questions according to what has been most consistently true over your child's lifetime, then tally your selections and record the number of responses for each in the spaces below. For questions that may have more than one applicable answer, simply select the statement that most closely identifies your child's main attributes. Let the journey begin!

1. I would describe my child as . . .
   a. quick and restless
   b. sharp and aggressive
   c. calm and steady

2. When it comes to remembering things, my child . . .
   a. tends to forget almost immediately
   b. retains a fair amount of what is absorbed
   c. easily retains, recollects, and remembers

3. Thoughts running through my child's head are . . .
   a. constantly changing
   b. fairly consistent
   c. always steady and stable

4. My child is able to concentrate . . .
    a. for short periods of time, but is easily distracted
    b. in moderate stretches, with determination
    c. for considerably long periods of time

5. When my child is learning something new, they grasp it . . .
    a. almost instantly
    b. adequately, but may take some time
    c. very slowly, often with difficulty

6. If my child's dreams were a movie, they would feature . . .
    a. fear, dread, running, jumping
    b. adventure, violence, anger, fire
    c. friends, lots of water, and clouds

7. My child's sleep pattern is . . .
    a. usually interrupted with a lot of tossing and turning
    b. mostly peaceful
    c. deep and heavy, doesn't wake easily

8. The term that best describes my child's speech . . .
    a. the local metro – fast, unclear, often skips or fumbles words
    b. the bullet train – fast, but clear and well thought out
    c. the luxury cruise – slow, clear, and sweet

9. When my child speaks, it usually comes out in this fashion . . .
    a. high-pitched
    b. medium-pitched
    c. low-pitched

10. When I serve my child's favorite meal, they . . .
    a. race to the table and quickly clear the plate
    b. eat at a moderate speed
    c. savor every bite at a leisurely pace

11. My child gets hungry . . .
    a. very often
    b. irregularly
    c. not often

12. My child's favorite meals and beverages are . . .
    a. wonderfully warm soups, stews, and hot cocoa
    b. cold fruit and veggies, cool drinks and treats
    c. warm crunchy, munchy snacks . . . popcorn is a favorite!

13. When it comes to achieving goals, my child is . . .
    a. easily distracted and flighty
    b. unstoppable and competitive
    c. slow and steady to the finish line

14. In school, my child works most efficiently . . .
    a. under supervision
    b. alone, at their own pace
    c. working as part of a group or team

15. The kind of weather that most irritates my child is . . .
    a. a cold morning
    b. a hot afternoon
    c. a damp, cool day

16. When the going gets tough, my child . . .
    a. gets easily stressed, wants to leave
    b. feels slightly intimidated, but perseveres
    c. stays calm, doesn't get worked up

17. Friends, friends, friends . . .
    a. quite a lot, although most are short-term
    b. my child is a bit of a loner
    c. only a couple, but special ones who have been around for a long time

18. When it comes to mood swings, my child . . .
    a. changes lanes faster than a sports car
    b. holds steady for a while, then fluctuates
    c. remains steady and stable

19. My child's number one defense mechanism when it comes to stress is . . .
    a. to have an emotional outburst
    b. to become angry and critical
    c. none, they are calm

20. My child has a soft side for . . .
    a. depends on the day
    b. nothing in particular
    c. people's feelings

21. If I told my child our family was moving to a new town, they would . . .
    a. run away crying and crawl into a favorite hiding spot
    b. yell and scream and fight
    c. calmly ask for details and ways to help out

22. My child expresses affection toward people they love . . .
    a. with a handwritten poem, letter, or craft
    b. with a shiny new gift
    c. with great emotion and lots of hugs

23. I can tell my child is hurt when they . . .
    a. cry a river
    b. needlessly argue
    c. lock themselves in their room

24. My child's instant reaction to an emotional trauma like a lost doll or treasured possession is . . .
    a. anxiety
    b. denial
    c. depression

25. The following situation that best describes my child's confidence level . . .
    a. hardly looks new friends in the eye
    b. can easily talk to a group of children about any topic, new or old
    c. can step up when the situation demands, but takes great effort

26. My child's hair is . . .
    a. dry as a desert
    b. normal
    c. very oily

27. My child's natural hair color is . . .
    a. light brown/blond
    b. red/auburn
    c. dark brown/black

28. I'd categorize my child's skin type as . . .
    a. dry, rough, maybe both
    b. soft, normal, maybe a little oily
    c. cool, moist, oily

29. When it comes to body temperature, my child . . .
    a. always has cold hands, makes frequent requests to turn up the heat
    b. runs warm, likes the windows open all year
    c. feels pleasantly cool, not too hot, not too cold

30. My child's complexion within our own ethnicity is . . .
    a. on the darker side, tans easily
    b. pinkish or reddish
    c. fairer and/or pale

31. My child's eyes are . . .
    a. small
    b. normal
    c. large

32. The whites of my child's eyes are . . .
    a. blue/brown
    b. yellow/red
    c. glossy white

33. My child's wide smile is made of . . .
    a. small teeth
    b. small to medium teeth
    c. medium to large teeth

34. Judging by my child's weight, they would feel right at home with the . . .
    a. lightweight society
    b. medium-weight bunch
    c. heavy-weight league

35. My child's bowel movements are . . .
    a. dry and hard, easily constipated
    b. soft to normal, several times a day
    c. heavy and thick, may take extra time in the bathroom

a: _____ b: _____ c: _____

a = Vata b = Pitta c = Kapha

INTERPRETING YOUR CHILD'S SCORE

Now that you have the total scores of your child's prakriti quiz for vata, pitta, and kapha, you can identify your child's constitution according to the ratio of the doshas. It is normal to have some numbers in all three sections as there are seven different possible combinations for an Ayurvedic constitution. Single types are vata, pitta, kapha. Dual types are vata-pitta, vata-kapha, pitta-kapha. The tridoshic type, which is quite rare, is vata-pitta-kapha. Your final assessment should be based on comparing the most prominent scores that identify and reflect the qualities and characteristics of the doshas. Please follow the criteria here to discover your child's prakriti.

a	b	c	Constitution
>14	<11	<11	Vata
<11	>14	<11	Pitta
<11	<11	>14	Kapha
>12	>12	<10	Vata-Pitta
>12	<10	>12	Vata-Kapha
<10	>12	>12	Pitta-Kapha
>10	>10	>10	Vata-Pitta-Kapha

Knowing your child's prakriti allows you to see the different influences the three doshas have on your children and gives you another tool to keep everyday life in balance. The results of the quiz you just took will help you better understand your children's mental and physical strengths and weaknesses along with their tendencies and affinities so you can put the art and science of the Ayurvedic lifestyle to work—the key to prevention. You may have already identified specific tendencies or habits in your children throughout this chapter that correlate to the three doshas, and no doubt you will discover many more as you continue to explore your child's constitution. Not only will this knowledge support you to create and adjust your child's daily wellness routines to keep the doshas in balance, but it also gives you a baseline from which you can recognize and correct imbalances that arise.

Being attuned to your child's constitution not only allows you to strive for optimal health throughout all the stages of childhood using the lifestyle tools you discover throughout this book, but also is the best way to create multidimensional daily routines that support your child's physical, mental, and spiritual well-being. Next, we'll take a look at the ways kapha dosha influences the age of childhood and how to best support your child's immunity.

3

SUPPORTING CHILDHOOD IMMUNITY

IF YOU HAVE ever thought about natural ways to boost your child's immune system ahead of cold and flu season or before returning to a classroom full of germs when the new school year begins, you're right in step with the Ayurvedic view. Ayurveda's natural healing principles understand that immunity is within us, and we can support and enhance our own immune resistance. In fact, the very definition of immunity in Ayurveda is the ability of the body to resist and overcome any disease process. Immunity depends on how balanced and strong your system is so that it can resist imbalances like viruses and bacteria. When your immune system is robust, pathogens won't be able to intrude and create disease. We can also look at immunity and everyday health issues with our newfound understanding of the doshas and see how to balance them before we get into the basics of everyday care. As Ayurveda gains popularity as a holistic life science alongside other types of complementary and mind-body medicine, more and more families are turning to natural remedies to boost immunity and manage everyday health issues—especially when it comes to their children.

The Age of Kapha

Now that you have discovered your child's individual prakriti, let's zoom out for a moment and take a broader perspective of the overarching kapha age of childhood.

If you've ever felt like you're a human sneeze guard or endlessly in search of a tissue to mop up your child's runny nose, there's a reason for that! According to Ayurveda, kapha reigns supreme during childhood, and the various qualities of the kapha dosha are expressed more predominately during this time of life. Since every child is governed by the kapha dosha, there is a greater tendency toward kapha-related health issues. By nature, kapha is heavy, sticky, and slow. As you probably know from your own experience, the accumulation of these qualities leads to coughs, colds, earaches, upper respiratory infections, allergies, and—of course—lots of excess mucus. Recognizing some of the common pitfalls associated with childhood that often lead to illness can help you fend off and manage a good number of those coughs and colds in your home.

You may be wondering where this fits in to balancing the doshas according to your child's prakriti. Shouldn't that be enough to prevent any imbalances that might lead to these common illnesses? Yes—if it weren't for the fact that the doshas continuously shift both within you and around you in your external environments. Since it is impossible to synchronously balance what is always in motion, the key to prevention is recognizing signs of imbalance and aggravation before the seeds of illness take root and manifest as a disease or disorder that becomes harder and more complicated to treat.

The same way you experience various daily imbalances from an interrupted night's sleep, changes in the weather, eating on the go, or simply through the course of a day's emotional highs and lows, your children also cycle through the dynamic balancing act of the doshas—except they don't feel or express these subtle changes in their bodies the same way you do as an adult and aren't yet fully capable of taking the necessary steps to correct them. This is where you come in. Without your awareness and intervention, these imbalances will require a much longer time for the body to correct on its own and leave your children vulnerable to further aggravation and illnesses.

In the same way parenthood challenges you to continuously foster your children's positive behavior, development, and enthusiasm and curiosity for life, your commitment to their health is the single most important influence on your child's well-being. Your close attention can support your children beyond measure during this vital stage and, no less important, show them the ways to live in harmony with nature and how to respect their unique constitution throughout their lives. From toddler to teen, Ayurveda offers you a path that can deeply nurture and renew your relationships with your children and at the same time awaken the joys of mindfulness practices within you. It starts with simple, quiet observation of your child's expressions.

Just as important as striving for balance to maintain your child's health is understanding the ways to gently restore imbalances when they do arise—as they will. There are a few variables you should be aware of that may require a little more attention. For example, if you have a kapha child who is already prone to kapha disorders, the age of childhood itself presents another contributing factor that can increase tendencies of a kapha imbalance. Similarly, the kapha-dominant seasons of late winter and spring add yet another layer of instability. You can see the ways that simply being aware of different influences in your children's environments can help you adjust their lifestyle routines accordingly. As the saying goes, an ounce of prevention is worth a pound of cure—the cornerstone of Ayurvedic principles.

The good news—the great news actually—is that imbalances that occur during the kapha stage of life are the easiest to correct since this stage represents nourishment and stability. During this period marked by rapid growth and development, the ratio of nourishment outpaces degeneration and naturally supports healing and regeneration compared to the other life stages marked by the fire and transformation of pitta and the movement and dryness of vata. A little of your support during this period in life goes a long way toward minimizing your child's symptoms and suffering and allows you to restore balance quite easily.

Immunity

According to Ayurveda, every individual possesses all the healing mechanisms necessary within every system of the body to both resist and recover from health problems. In other words—everyone has the tools for robust immunity. When you support the immune system naturally, rather than suppress it, you can strengthen your child's innate resistance to imbalances and build a powerful first line of defense.

Let's examine how this works using the example of increasingly prevalent seasonal allergies—a common culprit for children suffering from symptoms of allergic rhinitis at the same time every year. Why is your child sneezing, sniffling, and possibly even wheezing or having difficulty breathing while other children are happily running around enjoying the bloom of spring? The standard response is to blame the seasonal pollens wafting through the air from trees, weeds, and grasses. But the reality is that if the pollens were really the problem, every child exposed would suffer the same way. It's actually not the pollen at all, but a hyperactive immune response that makes certain children reactive and symptomatic to these exposures. It would be challenging to zero in on exactly why your child is hypersensitive to certain allergens as there are many factors that contribute to hypersensitivity of the immune system including genetics, diet and lifestyle, and sensory, emotional, and mental inputs. Ayurveda's approach to these types of conditions is to stabilize and strengthen the immune system and carefully manage diet and lifestyle routines to reduce exposures and return the body to a state of balance.

Let's take a look at what happens to the immune system when you give your child an over-the-counter antihistamine or decongestant—after all, you don't want your children to suffer, and allergies can interfere with everything from sleep to schoolwork, leaving kids miserable and exhausted. While it's true that OTC allergy medications may offer some immediate symptomatic relief, they can never provide a long-term sustainable outcome—the most important factor for your children. Relying on these products leads to greater exposure to the allergens, recurrent inflammation, and a higher likelihood of developing chronic degenerative changes in the respiratory system. In addition to the unwanted side effects many of these products can cause such as drowsiness and dullness, giving your child OTC medications for symptomatic relief works directly against the body's natural defense mechanisms. For example, coughing and sneezing are the body's protective responses to expel the allergens creating a crisis in the lungs. The wheezing and difficulty breathing that sometimes follow are a result of the body's natural response to constrict the lungs and minimize exposure of the irritating allergens. Ayurveda's approach to managing immunity issues is to strengthen and stabilize the immune system and reduce hypersensitivity reactions so the body's innate defense mechanisms remain uncompromised and can resist possible irritations and inflammation.

When it comes to keeping your child's immune system strong and resilient, a good defense truly is the best offense. In parts two and three of this book, we will discuss the many different Ayurvedic tools and techniques you can follow to maintain your child's health and keep the doshas balanced, including diet and lifestyle routines, herbal formulations and applications, yoga, meditation, therapeutic Ayurvedic oil massage, breathing exercises, and even sound therapy. Later, you will find basic recipes to enhance your child's immunity along with simple home remedies for common childhood complaints in chapter 16.

Let's look next at some useful Ayurvedic tools that can help you manage common immunity-related conditions and get your children on the road to recovery as quickly as possible.

Immunity-Related Conditions

Many parents feel like their children have only just recovered from one bout of something when they get struck with another. For busy parents, waging war against the steady stream of germs running through the house can feel like a losing battle. Following some basic Ayurvedic tips lets you manage your child's symptoms like a pro, cut back on missed days of school, and catch up on some much-needed rest yourself.

COLDS AND CONGESTION

Let's talk first about colds and congestion—by far the most common immunity-related conditions your children are likely to experience over and over . . . and over again! First and foremost, avoid any exposure to cold. This includes foods, beverages, and even weather—and at the top of that list is ice. We will take a deeper look at the ways ice and cold drinks extinguish your child's digestive fire according to the Ayurvedic principle of *agni* in chapter 5, but for now just know that ice in any form—including the ice you blend into your child's favorite smoothie—is crucial to avoid until symptoms abate. For children especially prone to congestion, including recurring ear infections, it is best to follow these guidelines as often as possible, especially during the kapha-predominant seasons of late winter and spring. When you do venture outside into the cold together to play or send your children to school, remember to protect them as much as possible by bundling them up in warm clothing and outerwear that will keep their extremities warm.

The second tip for managing colds at home is to minimize hair washing. According to Ayurveda, wetting the scalp is a common trigger for congestion, which suggests you reduce the frequency of this routine. You can still give your child a warm, comforting bath or shower once or twice a day, but limiting the frequency of hair washing just may ward off that next cold. The general rule of thumb is to limit washing your child's hair to once a week or so if they have a tendency toward congestion and refrain from wetting the head at all when your child is suffering from symptoms of colds or congestion. When you do wash your child's hair, be sure to thoroughly towel-dry the scalp or use a mild blow-dryer setting. Also take care to avoid extreme heat as Ayurveda considers this exposure unhealthy for the hair and eyes.

As parents know better than anyone, feeding a sick child can be tricky business. Very often, appetites run low, and a cranky mood can leave your child pickier than ever when it comes to mealtimes. According to Ayurveda, food is nature's medicine and has tremendous power to heal, support, nourish, and repair when consumed properly. You should consider what you offer your children to eat throughout the course of an illness vital to their recovery. Your food choices can either pacify imbalances or further aggravate them, resulting in greater accumulation and imbalance of congestion in this case. This can lead to worsening symptoms, unnecessary OTC interventions, frequent visits to the doctor, and repeated antibiotic use. We will examine Ayurvedic nutritional guidelines more closely in chapter 4 and discuss the ins and outs of what to feed your children, but the most important recommendation when it comes to colds and congestion is to offer your child easily digestible, cooked food and hold off on the raw veggies and salads until recovery is complete. It is also best to refrain from anything oily and too many sweets.

Remember, the best way to support your child's colds and congestion and shorten the duration of illness is through warmth. Keep an eye on the thermostat, be at the ready with a warm sweater and extra blankets, and offer your child plenty of warm water and herbal teas to sip throughout the day. And don't overlook the importance of those warming cuddles and hugs!

ALLERGIES

If you've ever been advised to keep your kids indoors and the windows shut on a breezy spring day when pollen counts are high, chances are you have a child who suffers from allergies. Maybe you've heeded this advice in the past—or tried to, at least, but were moved by the feeling that there must be a better solution. Keeping your children from going outside to play and enjoying the blossoming spring flowers and warmer days seems detrimental in other ways and an unfair punishment on top of all the sneezing, coughing, and sniffling they endure from the hallmark symptoms of allergic rhinitis. With allergies on the rise for millions of children, more parents than ever are looking for ways to prevent and effectively treat the symptoms of seasonal allergies.

As mentioned earlier, Ayurveda identifies allergies as hypersensitivity of the body's immune system. In other words, it's not about the allergens or the pollen—or even the season. It's about the strength and stability of your child's immune system. The remedy isn't to keep them from playing outside, it is to enhance your child's immunity.

Ayurveda takes a comprehensive approach to managing seasonal allergies that considers your child's body, mind, and environment. Treatment begins with minimizing exposures to specific allergens while supporting your child's immune resistance, then slowly reintroducing specific environmental triggers. This process involves careful management of your child's diet, routines, and mental exposures along with the use of immunity-stabilizing herbs that an experienced Ayurvedic physician can recommend as part of a comprehensive treatment protocol.

One of the best ways you can support your child's immune system naturally is using traditional household spices such as turmeric and ginger in small quantities when you are preparing food or teas. These are common kitchen spices that you may already have in your cabinet or are easily picked up at your local grocery store. One very effective home remedy to treat allergies, for example, is a simple preparation of turmeric powder with warm milk your child consumes daily for a few weeks. You will learn more about the effective uses and healing properties of herbs and spices when we discuss Ayurvedic nutrition, but in the meantime, you can find immunity-enhancing home recipes for common childhood conditions in chapter 16. Remember to follow the same kapha-reducing guidelines you would for colds and congestion if you have a child who suffers from allergies and take special care to avoid cold foods and beverages.

DAIRY, GLUTEN, AND OTHER FOOD SENSITIVITIES

With rapidly expanding gluten- and dairy-free aisles in your local grocery store and so many parents declaring their children are on restricted diets, it can be hard not to wonder if you should restock your pantry shelves at home and adapt to a new diet and lifestyle that might offer increased benefits to your children.

The primary reason for the gluten-free trend is that some children as well as adults develop intolerances to gluten ingredients. Food intolerances are hyperimmune sensitivities just as we have discussed with seasonal allergies, but some can be life-threatening and may need emergency management. In this case, the immune system identifies gluten as toxic and releases antibodies that create inflammation and lead to intestinal symptoms that can include bloating, excessive gas, cramps, nausea, diarrhea, and incomplete evacuation. This affects absorption of nutrients and overall nourishment. The only way to treat this issue is to strengthen and stabilize the child's immune system so it stops triggering the false alarm. It's the same with other food sensitivities such as dairy, for example.

While there are many children who are in fact intolerant to gluten and dairy products, these are person-specific, and there is no need for a universal approach to any type of diet or to avoid gluten or dairy without a reason. If you discover your child is allergic to gluten or dairy, at that point you can avoid those ingredients and create a protocol with an Ayurvedic professional to strengthen and stabilize their immune system against the sensitivity and carefully reintroduce the ingredients slowly over time.

Allergies and intolerances take many forms from babies who are allergic to their mother's breast milk to sudden, adult-onset food sensitivities. Regardless of age or type of hypersensitivity, here is a good step-by-step approach:

1. Avoid items known to create allergic reactions in the body, whether it is milk, wheat, rice, or breast milk.
2. Guide diet and lifestyle practices based on age, constitution, and type of allergies.
3. Integrate specific Ayurveda and yoga health enhancement practices into your child's routines, such as regular *neti* (nasal irrigation), *nasya* (nasal drops), *pranayama* (breathing practices), *asana* (body postures), meditation, *abhyanga* (massage with oil), and so on.
4. Consider condition-specific and immunity-enhancing herbs and herbal formulations under the guidance of an Ayurvedic practitioner with the goal to stabilize and strengthen immune resistance against allergens for at least a few months.
5. Follow a course of *panchakarma* (Ayurvedic purification process) followed by *rasayanas* (rejuvenating protocol) under the supervision of an Ayurvedic doctor if the individual requires such a healing process and is eligible based on considerations like age and condition of health.
6. Monitor the condition and reassess the individual's health based on Ayurvedic principles on a periodic basis.

7. Slowly reintroduce the items that caused sensitivities once the individual is stable and stronger as per the Ayurvedic assessment.

ECZEMA AND PSORIASIS

While allergies are the hypersensitivity of the immune system to something outside of the body, eczema and psoriasis are the hypersensitivity of the immune system to its own tissues and systems. These types of conditions cause your immune system to mistake your body's own healthy cells and tissues as foreign and attack as if they were pathogens. This is known as autoimmunity. Since this is another type of aberration of the immune system, strengthening your child's immune system will provide the best sustainable, long-term outcome.

In addition to boosting immunity, there are certain dietary triggers you'll want to avoid or minimize because they can increase the irritation and itching associated with eczema-related skin disorders. These include anything that creates sliminess in the system such as yogurt, sour oranges, mangoes, vinegars, and even sesame seeds. Preparing warm, freshly cooked foods, reducing sweets, and monitoring your child's dairy intake can correct primary imbalances that lead to eczema and psoriasis.

With the many benefits you can achieve by following Ayurveda's nutritional guidelines, it can be easy to overlook your child's lifestyle routines. Is your child staying up too late at night or not getting enough exercise? Ayurveda's recommendations for eliminating and reducing symptoms of these autoimmune conditions and providing supportive care emphasize both a kapha-balancing diet *and* lifestyle. Be mindful of your child's routines and activity levels, and bear in mind happiness is very much a part of healthiness! Keep your children's spirits high by visiting new places and varying your local adventures and activities with them to stimulate excitement and curiosity.

Parents often want to know how long it will take for symptoms to resolve once they begin following various Ayurvedic remedies and protocols. Natural approaches to systemic conditions may require some time to see results. Remember, Ayurveda addresses the root causes of all disease and disorders and strives to eliminate underlying imbalances. When you only treat health symptoms, you will see conditions manifest again and again and often progress into a chronic ailment or disorder. That said, as imbalances start to correct, you will begin to notice that your child's flare-ups become less frequent or perhaps don't require management as often with steroid creams or antihistamines, for example. The body expresses healing just as it expresses disease. Stay tuned in to your child's mind-body expressions, remain adaptable to modifying lifestyle protocols as needed, and always express a positive outlook—your energy plays a vital role in your child's recovery!

PART TWO

The Four Inputs

FOOD, WATER, BREATH, AND PERCEPTION

4

FOOD

IF YOU'RE LIKE most parents, knowing which nutritional guidelines to follow today in a sea of contradictory dietary advice, fad diets, and long lists of foods to avoid—that sometimes exclude entire food groups—can make mealtime feel downright messy. The last thing you want to do after a busy day when it's time to put dinner on the table is second-guess your food choices. To make matters worse, parents often worry they are doing more harm than good and depriving their children of a myriad of health benefits by not following the latest popular advice and nutritional trends—adding one more concern to your plate.

The modern parent ends up puzzled. Is the apple you're about to cut up for your child's snack chock-full of the same nutrients as the organic apple you could have bought if you had time to go to your local farmer's market or a different grocery store? Why is everyone suddenly gluten-free and lactose intolerant? Should you stop giving your child milk? Will one of the dozens of nondairy milk alternatives provide your children the protein and nutrients they need? Throw in the prevalence of childhood allergies and various conditions along with an abundance of superfoods and supplements available on today's market, and it may feel like you've just lost the helm of your grocery cart. There must be an easier way to view food and nutrition. And in fact, there is.

The Four Inputs

Now that you have discovered Ayurveda's fundamental principles of keeping the doshas balanced and fluently in sync with nature, it's time to uncover the four inputs (*ahara*) that nurture, nourish, and maintain the flow of life: food, water, breath, and perception, which we'll cover throughout the next four chapters. Ayurveda views human existence as a true microcosm of the universe at large and poetically explains that life is like a perennial river, continuously flowing and symbolizing the course of life itself. A river starts on a mountain cliff as a small stream, then runs downward through the valley, joining other channels of water to form larger streams, deepening and widening until it reaches the end of its passage, finally merging with the ocean. In the same way, human life starts as a single cell in the mother's womb and continues to multiply until a human being emerges to grow and develop in the flow of life's journey. That life continues to flow, inseparable from nature, until it eventually disintegrates and merges with the universe. Along the way, the body undergoes many processes of degeneration and deterioration of cells, bodily tissues, and the energy we use for various physical and mental functions required for day-to-day activities and development. For regeneration and replenishment to optimally occur, a constant systematic inflow is necessary to maintain this river of life.

The food that nourishes your children's bodies, for example, also has the power to nourish their minds and souls when consumed according to body constitution and the Ayurvedic nutritional guidelines we are about to explore. Water consumption not only replenishes lost fluids, but it also aids digestion and absorption and strengthens or weakens the system's agni, or metabolism. From your child's very first breath, each and every inhalation and exhalation carries *prana* or life energy, throughout all the subtle energy channels of the system and connects the body and mind. Inhalations energize, stabilize, and nurture whereas exhalations purify and detoxify. Finally, perception determines how the internal self receives various stimuli from the outside world through the five senses. The mind's entire framework for the way your children see, hear, touch, and respond to every piece of information they encounter in life relies on the input of perception.

When you view human existence as inseparable from nature and the influences of your changing environment the same way a river is inseparable from the universe, you can help chart your child's journey according to Ayurveda's four inputs of life and set them on a path to express their highest potential.

Food: The Primary Input

According to Ayurveda, food is the first and primary of the four inputs of life and ensures your child's health, vitality, growth, and development. This includes proper nourishment of organs and tissues, development of sensory acuity, and balanced function of all the body systems. Did you know your child's overall vitality is the collective outcome of well-nourished tissues and balanced digestion and metabolism? Your food choices determine your child's present and long-term vitality. This is known as *ojas* in Ayurveda and is synonymous with vibrancy, vitality, immune strength, and sustainable energy. Ojas is the supreme glow of the body expressed as an outcome of optimal nourishment of all the tissues. And when we talk about vitality in Ayurveda, it includes physical strength, digestive and metabolic strength, sustainable energy, immune resistance, and the overall vibrance of an individual—vibrance not only in the physical sense but in an individual's ability to focus and learn, remember and retrieve information (memory recall), and feel calm and balanced.

According to Kaumarabhritya, food is the primary ingredient that facilitates the growth and development of your child, and it considers incorporation of various principles of nutrition crucial—both to prevent and manage many of today's most prevalent pediatric conditions. Have you ever heard the saying "food is medicine"? Food has tremendous healing capacities and supports your body's innate intelligence to resist and treat various diseases and disorders. Here are just a few examples: Winter melon heals degenerative lung conditions and manages anxiety. Arrowroot powder heals the gut. Black raisins heal anemia. Wild Indian yams heal hemorrhoids. Cumin and ginger relieve indigestion and bloating, and coriander seed heals urinary complications.

Ayurveda makes it easy for parents to follow simple nutritional guidelines that will nourish your child's mind, body, and soul and encourage you to rely more on your own intuition at mealtimes and less on the latest and greatest nutritional study subject to dramatic patterns. No calorie counting necessary.

Three Ayurvedic Principles of Nutrition

There are three factors Ayurveda primarily considers when it comes to food: what to eat, how much to eat, and when to eat. Which one of these do you think is the most important? It may come as a surprise to people accustomed to Western diet principles that *when* to eat assumes the highest priority. Let's look at the science.

WHEN TO EAT

Every single function within your body—and the entirety of nature—is regulated by cyclical rhythms like sunrise and sunset, lunar rhythms, and seasonal rhythms. The same way everything in nature is cyclical, every function of the human mind-body system also works in cyclic rhythms— the cardiac rhythm, the respiratory rhythm, the digestive rhythm, the sleep rhythm, and the menstrual rhythm, for example. Even biochemical changes take place in cyclical rhythms such as enzymatic cycles, sugar cycles, and hormone cycles.

Ayurvedic principles show that if you are able to follow a regular eating pattern and establish breakfast, lunch, and dinnertime routines, over time that regularly repeated message will result in a circadian consciousness within your mind-body system. This in turn allows digestive secretions, enzymes, and hormones to seamlessly support the entire digestive process for optimal assimilation, absorption, and utilization of nutrients. The human body has an amazing intelligence superior to that of our minds in many ways, leaving us with much less to do than we imagine—which is always good news for parents!

You may be wondering how you can maintain consistent mealtimes if you have school-age children who have assigned eating periods that are beyond your control. It is important to do your best on the mealtimes you do have a say over at home in that case because, knowingly or unknowingly, a general rhythm will naturally set in for your children depending on what time they need to leave the house in the morning and the particular time they are scheduled to eat lunch each day. Your conscious awareness of these rhythms will help support your child's nourishment, vitality, and energy levels.

How long exactly does it take to establish this consciousness within your child's system—especially one that may have already gone haywire? According to Ayurveda, when you continue something at a particular time each day for one lunar cycle—or twenty-eight days—your system will become attuned to that schedule. It only takes twenty-eight days to reset your child's entire system? Yes—and yours too if you wish, as the same principle applies to adults.

Let's take a look next at what happens physiologically when you don't pay attention to maintaining your children's eating schedule. First, let's consider a couple of statistics. One out of three children and adolescents in the United States are either overweight or suffering from childhood obesity, and the percentage of children affected by obesity has more than tripled since the 1970s. Metabolic imbalances are unquestionably on the rise. Establishing a cyclical rhythm of eating for children can help diminish these tendencies.

How exactly do regular mealtimes reduce your child's chances of developing a metabolic disorder? All of the food you eat gets utilized in three ways. First, your body absorbs glucose and directly transforms it into energy. Second, food can be utilized for tissue nourishment—the most important for children as they are in a rapid growth stage of life, a time when their muscles, bones, nerves, and all of their tissues need to be continually nourished. Third, any leftover balance is deposited as fat for crisis management. When you maintain a mealtime schedule and establish a consistent rhythm of eating, your entire system is ready to digest, absorb, and utilize all the food you ingest. As a result, there is little chance of having any unwanted accumulation of unutilized food. According to Ayurveda, every metabolic disorder is defined simply by that which is not completely and properly transformed. When there is little or no balance left over from the food you eat, your chances of developing a metabolic disorder will be very minimal as that excess accumulation is what can lead to metabolic disorders such as obesity and diabetes.

Often, in India, Dr. J would encounter distressed mothers who sought out pediatric care because their children weren't eating. One woman from a remote village in Bangalore traveled with her four-year-old boy, saying he had barely eaten anything for days. In consultation it became clear the child was not being offered meals according to any kind of schedule and was instead randomly snacking on candy and other sugary treats—then refusing to eat any semblance of a normal meal. Dr. J advised the mother to monitor her son's candy intake and to feed him only at specific mealtimes. The woman was certain she needed an Ayurvedic herbal formulation to support her child, so Dr. J also recommended digestive drops, promising they would work as soon as she started feeding her child at regular times each day. Soon afterward, a second woman from the same village arrived at Dr. J's with her own son in tow, asking for the same magic herbs that had helped her friend's child! Of course it was simply the rhythm of established mealtimes that had effectively treated the problem.

WHAT TO EAT

The second principle in Ayurvedic nutrition discusses the key points in deciding *what* to eat. Fundamentally, children have different nutritional needs based on age, constitution, and nutritional requirements due to activity levels, which are assessed in terms of how a child spends their day and how physically or minimally active they are overall. Obviously, a very athletic child needs more food than a less active one. Moving beyond these basic considerations, Ayurveda looks at the most important factor in determining every type of lifestyle or treatment plan for every person—individual constitution, or prakriti.

According to Ayurveda and as we've discovered in chapter 2, every individual is born with a certain innate nature that will remain the same throughout a person's lifetime—similar to the concept of DNA. Ayurveda classifies these body constitutions into seven different types, meaning if you take all of the children on the planet they can be categorized into one of seven groups based on their mind-body nature. According to that nature, your child's tendencies and affinities will vary—and so should their diet.

A kapha child, for example, has a natural tendency to gain weight and experience accumulation. These children want to limit heavier foods and opt for a lighter diet, whereas children with a vata constitution tend to be dry, lean, and emaciated and require more nourishing and oily types of foods. In the same way, the warm and sharp qualities of pitta call for a more cooling, grounding diet. When you assess your child's dosha along with current imbalances, you can easily gain an understanding of which foods will pacify and support your child's constitution. These three elements together—age, constitution, and activity levels—can help you determine a blueprint for meal planning based on food choices that will support optimal nutrition as well as prevent, manage, and minimize recurrence of disorders and disease.

This brings us to one of the key principles of balancing the doshas through an Ayurvedic diet. Parents often wonder if they should focus on constitution or a specific imbalance when deciding what their children should eat. According to Ayurveda, the primary focus should always be to correct any imbalance first. Once the imbalance has been corrected, you can continue to follow nutritional guidelines for your child's constitution. Simply put, when there is an imbalance, focus on the imbalance; when there is no imbalance, focus on the constitution.

THE AYURVEDIC BALANCED MEAL

After hours of precious downtime spent every week planning meals, parents are still looking for an answer to the million-dollar question—what exactly constitutes an ideal balanced meal?

Ayurveda considers a balanced meal to be a wholesome blend of food based on the *principle of the six tastes*. Ayurveda explains that all foods contain one or a multiple of the tastes sweet, sour, salty, pungent, astringent, and bitter, and each taste has its own distinct functional effects on the mind-body system as indicated in the charts on the following pages. Different tastes impact the mind and body according to which ones are most predominant in your diet. The inverse is also true—too little or less than is required of one or more tastes can also lead to imbalances.

As you know, children generally crave a lot of sweets, but what you might not know is this is actually considered a requirement in the growing stage of life because sweet is the most nourishing of the six tastes. Caution: when we say *sweet* in Ayurvedic terms, this doesn't mean sugar as in lollipops and cake—it also includes grains, milk, rice, lentils, chicken, and other foods you can find on the Six Tastes Chart here.

Six Tastes Chart

Taste	Elemental Composition	Examples
Sweet	Earth + Water	Dates, raisins, sugar, jaggery, rice, potato
Sour	Earth + Fire	Lemon, lime, vinegar, tomato, yogurt
Salty	Water + Fire	Sea salt, Himalayan pink salt, black salt
Pungent	Fire + Air	Cayenne pepper, ginger, black pepper, jalapeños
Astringent	Air + Earth	Pomegranate peel, kale, unripe persimmon
Bitter	Air + Space	Bitter melon, dandelion, cocoa, aloe

Influence of Tastes on Doshas

DOSHA	Supporting Tastes	Tastes to be Reduced/Avoided	Positive Desire for Tastes	Imbalanced Craving
Vata	Sweet, sour, and salty	Bitter, pungent, and astringent	Sweet, sour, and salty	Pungent, astringent, and bitter
Pitta	Sweet, astringent, and bitter	Pungent, sour, and salty	Sweet, astringent, and bitter	Sour, salty, and pungent
Kapha	Pungent, astringent, and bitter	Sweet, sour, and salty	Pungent, astringent, and bitter	Sweet, sour, and salty

Other tastes important for children are sour, salty, and a little bit pungent, which are considered facilitators for digestion and absorption. Lastly, we come to the bitter and astringent tastes that are used sparingly when preparing food for children as these two tastes are reductive, drying, and depleting.

This Ayurvedic principle simply states that a proper blend of all six tastes constitutes a balanced meal. You will find that such a plate contains the necessary requirements of protein, fat, and carbohydrates your child needs for proper growth and development. Once you begin serving meals that contain an adequate amount of grains, protein, vegetables, and fruit, you can also use some household kitchen spices to enhance your child's digestion. Common spices like turmeric, cumin, coriander, or a little bit of black pepper are all found to be very effective in supporting digestion. From this point, you can continue to fine-tune your children's individual diets according to other factors including digestive strength, season, weather, and current imbalances.

Keep in mind that all of the Ayurvedic principles on nutrition are supported by one simple guideline: follow a natural, wholesome meal plan with ingredients like whole grains, vegetables, fruits, lentils, and spices, and try to avoid or minimize processed, canned, preserved, and refined food items. The human body is a natural living entity and can easily digest, absorb, and utilize natural wholesome ingredients, whereas chemically processed, bleached, or refined ingredients create crisis in the body that leads to inflammation and various diseases.

Taste	Organs of Primary Influence	Tendency for Diseases Due to Indulgence of Tastes	Action on the Mind	Effect of Over-indulgence	Examples of Foods/Ingredients
Sweet	Spleen, pancreas	Diabetes, obesity, weak digestion	Compassion, satisfaction	Attachment, possessiveness	Complex carbohydrates, sweet fruits, grains, root vegetables such as potatoes and beets, sugar, milk, oils, meats
Sour	Small intestine	Infections, ulcers, bleeding disorders	Discrimination, stimulation	Envy, jealousy, anger	Yogurt, sour fruits, raw mango, alcohol, vinegar, cheese
Salty	Kidneys	Hypertension, fluid retention	Confidence, zest for life	Greed, over ambition	Rock salt, sea salt, black salts
Pungent	Lungs	Dry lungs, dry cough, bleeding	Extroversion, boldness	Anger, violence, hatred	Jalapeños, ginger, black pepper, cloves, cayenne pepper, garlic, wasabi (horseradish)
Astringent	Heart	Anemia, low blood pressure, insomnia	Introversion	Insecurity, fear	Peel of a fruit, unripe banana, pomegranate peel, leafy green vegetables, cranberries
Bitter	Colon	Constipation, gas, bloating	Dissatisfaction, isolation	Grief, sorrow	Leafy vegetables, aloe, fenugreek, black tea, bitter melon

One of the best things you can do for your children when it comes to their diet is avoid serving cold food and beverages, a primary cause of poor digestion. We will discuss this in more detail in the next chapter, but for now know that cold always causes constriction and stagnation. Ingesting cold food items weakens the digestive fire and may also increase congestion as well as any blockages that may be present in your child's body system. Warm food and beverages are always a better choice for your children and considered to be digestive enhancers that will improve circulation and boost your child's overall health.

Do you have kids that love raw vegetables or salads? That's great—and you don't have to banish your go-to cucumber slices, but a lot of raw veggies, which parents often think of as healthy, are actually difficult for the body to digest. Ayurveda simply suggests being mindful about how much raw food you give your children as all raw vegetables carry cold and dry qualities, which can hamper digestion and increase tendencies toward the colds and congestion your children are already prone to in this kapha stage of life. It is best to avoid raw items completely anytime you notice your child's digestion is dull or weak, which we'll cover shortly.

Digestion is a similar process to cooking. Just as the heat and flame of a stove can break down raw food ingredients into an easily digestible and absorbable form, the digestive secretions in your gut including salivary amylase, acids, and pepsin break down ingested food. Since the gut can only absorb nutritional ingredients like proteins, fats, or carbohydrates on a molecular level, it is much easier to absorb these nutrients from food that has already been broken down by cooking rather than raw food items.

This is a good point to address the popular notion that cooking vegetables destroys their nutritional value. The reality is that the natural proteins, fats, and carbohydrates of a particular food are never lost through cooking. It is true that some of the enzymes and vitamins can get denatured through cooking, but these are still abundant in fruit, which is considered much easier to digest than raw vegetables because the ripening process is equivalent to natural cooking. So you see, if you are providing balanced meals to your children, there is no need to worry about the minimal amount of nutrients that may be lost by cooking your broccoli when the fruit your child is eating will provide a regular, sufficient amount.

INCOMPATIBLE FOOD COMBINING

Ayurveda identifies and classifies food ingredients according to their unique properties, the six tastes, and individual health benefits along with the best practices of combining them properly to ensure optimal absorption and nourishment of all the body's systems and tissues. However, incompatible food combinations (*viruddha*) are also important to keep in mind. Ayurveda clearly states that certain food items cannot be combined with others because they can lead to health problems. These incompatibilities arise for various reasons such as incompatible potencies, opposite qualities, and improper interaction when consumed in the same quantities, to name a few. When you eat a meal with incompatible food combinations, it causes digestive imbalances along with metabolic and other systemic issues and aggravates the doshas. While it may not always be possible to follow these guidelines, it is best to become familiar with this table so you can avoid creating *ama*, or improperly digested food that may act as toxins, and other disturbances within your child's system. Following is a list of Ayurveda's key incompatible food combinations. It bears repeating that blending fruit with milk in the ever-popular fruit smoothie should be strongly avoided.

Food Ingredient	Incompatible with
Milk	Sour fruit, sour bread, fish, meat, yogurt, horse gram, jackfruit, radish, salt, moringa, lemon, lime, tamarind
Eggs	Yogurt, fruits, beans, cheese, and fish
Hot tea	Cold water
Fruits	Milk and yogurt

Food Ingredient	Incompatible with
Grains	Fruits
Honey	Equal quantity of ghee, radish, pork, never cook with honey or add to hot food or beverages
Radish	Milk, bananas, and raisins
Beans	Fruits, cheese, fish, milk, meat, yogurt, and eggs
Yogurt	Fruits, cheese, meat, milk, eggs, fish, chicken, banana
Black lentils	Monkey fruit, radish
Ghee	Equal quantity of honey, cold water or cold beverages
Meat	Milk, yogurt, cane jaggery, sesame seed, honey, black lentils, sprouts
Banana	Lentils, yogurt, radish
Cane jaggery	Radish, pork

HOW MUCH TO EAT

Portion control understandably receives a lot of attention in Western nutrition, as it is considered a key component in preventing and fighting obesity. The third component of the Ayurvedic nutrition principles explains the differences between Ayurvedic and conventional nutrition and will give you a different framework for planning your child's meals. How much should you eat? The answer of course is to eat in moderation, but outside of overeating or fasting, what exactly is moderation? It is the amount of food that nourishes your child without causing sluggishness in the digestive system or excessive accumulation. Since Ayurveda is person-specific, there is not a fixed quantity of food you should strive to serve your children. The best way to assess your child's nutritional needs and goals is to see how your child performs over a period of time. Do they have enough energy throughout the day? Are they gaining weight as expected? These types of considerations are the yardstick by which you can identify whether your child is overeating or undereating.

The modern approach to nutrition is based on two factors. One is the nutritional component of food—protein, carbohydrates, fat, and nutrients. The second is calories. Ayurveda has a much more comprehensive approach to nutrition and is not at all aligned with the concept of calorie counting. While Ayurveda agrees with the approach of monitoring input and output, the reality is that even when these match up—and despite controlling input in terms of calories and monitoring output in terms of activity—there is still a high incidence of diabetes and other metabolic disorders.

YOU ARE WHAT YOU DIGEST, NOT WHAT YOU EAT

There are many differences between conventional and Ayurvedic nutrition highlighted in the table here. According to Ayurveda, just because you eat something healthy, it doesn't mean your body will optimally digest and absorb all of the nutrients that food item has to offer and nourish your body. The general perception in modern nutrition is that if you are able to manage the quantity or intake of protein, carbohydrates, fats, vitamins, and minerals, you will be well-nourished. Hence the saying, *"You are what you eat."* Ayurveda has a different saying: *"You are what you digest."* There is a missing link in Western medicine that is Ayurveda's primary focus when it comes to nutrition: a person's internal digestive and metabolic efficiency.

When an individual's digestion and metabolism are weak, even minimal calorie intake can cause accumulation and lead to metabolic disorders like obesity due to poor transformation. Similarly, if your child's digestion and metabolism are strong and fast, even a slightly higher calorie intake than what may be standard will still not cause an accumulation because digestion and metabolism are burning bright and properly transforming calories. Ayurveda assigns much more importance to a person's internal digestive fire and metabolic efficiency than calorie computation—especially when it comes to children. Childhood is a time for growth, and you never want to inappropriately restrict calories during this period so crucial for nourishment and energy.

The Difference Between Conventional and Ayurvedic Nutrition

Subject	Conventional Nutrition	Ayurvedic Nutrition
Why We Eat	Personal preference, habit, body image, emotions, etc.	To take in prana to live
Nutritional Element	Calories	The five elements (Space, Air, Fire, Water, Earth)
Focus	Counting calories from the different food groups	How the body processes what we eat
Importance	Caloric value	Individual constitution
Balance	Balancing food ingredients	Balancing the diet according to prakriti
Dietary Recommendations	Depends on food groups	Depends on the six tastes of food
Slogan	You are what you eat.	You are what you digest.

In Dr. J's practice as an Ayurvedic physician over two decades, he has seen many children who eat the required amount of calories suggested by modern dietary nutritional guidelines yet still suffer from deficiencies, weaknesses, and depletion in their overall health in the forms of vitality, nourishment, and energy levels.

The efficiency of your child's digestive and metabolic system is what decides whether the food they eat will nourish them. It is by no means an absolute. You can eat all the food you want, but if it is not able to be properly digested, absorbed, and assimilated, it simply won't nourish the tissues because the body system isn't able to transform the food into nutrients. Keeping an eye on your child's digestive strength is key in making sure the food they eat will nourish them. We'll take a look at how to do that next and how to manage and improve digestive weaknesses.

MONITORING YOUR CHILD'S DIGESTION

How can you tell if your child has normal digestion? Natural methodologies are the best way to initially assess your child's digestive strength, and there are a few indicators parents can monitor that signal proper digestion. The first is that your child feels hungry and ready to eat at mealtimes. When your child has a strong appetite and asks for food at the usual times, it is an immediate indication that digestion is strong. Second is to monitor your child after mealtimes. Are there expressions of heaviness or tiredness? When digestion is weak, dullness impacts energy levels after a meal. The third is to ensure your child is properly tracking in weight gain and development. These are all indications of reasonably good digestion.

The first and foremost indication that your child's digestion is weak is a lack of interest in eating. It's much easier to monitor children than adults because they usually say what's on their mind, so if you're calling your child to the table at mealtimes and they are expressing disinterest in eating or aren't feeling hungry, this is when to really start watching for signals that their digestion may need a boost. Second is noticing that after eating a meal your child feels tired and wants to lie down or expresses they aren't feeling well. A decrease in activity after meals or sluggishness is also an indication of slow digestion. The third is if after eating a meal your child says their stomach hurts on a recurrent basis or feels nauseous or vomits. These are all indications of weak digestion.

Another scenario is when a child feels constantly hungry and eats a lot of food, but simply isn't gaining weight. The hunger is there, the quantity is there, but the nourishment and energy are not. This is also considered an indication of weak digestion because the tissues are craving nourishment. This tissue craving manifests as excessive hunger, but the digestion, absorption, and transformation of food into nutrients is not taking place. This is why despite having an appetite or even a heavy food intake, children sometimes don't get the nourishment they need. Ayurvedic principles state that proper digestion—not the quantity of food—is the primary source of proper nourishment. Efficiency is key.

Common Concerns about Modern Trends

Now that you know the three core principles of nutrition, you may be wondering where Ayurveda comes down on other nutrition trends as you consider sharing your own health practices with your child. What is the Ayurvedic take on vegetarian diets, vitamins, supplements, probiotics, and raw juicing?

PLANT-BASED AND VEGETARIAN DIETS

Should children follow a plant-based or vegetarian diet? Ayurveda classifies the properties and health benefits of all whole foods and natural ingredients found on the planet, so it is a myth that Ayurveda is strictly vegan or vegetarian. Ayurveda is a universal life science that believes individuals should follow their own beliefs and paths. Whether you wish to be a vegetarian or vegan is a deeply personal choice, and Ayurveda respects every person's individual practices. The overarching guidance is to follow healthy principles, avoid incompatible food combinations, and eat balanced meals in the right quantity at the right time.

VITAMINS, SUPPLEMENTS, AND PROBIOTICS

Many parents today who prioritize health and wellness or take supplements themselves wonder if they should be giving their children vitamins and supplements, especially with the myriad of options available on today's market. Ayurveda primarily suggests that if you prepare balanced, wholesome meals with a variety of fresh, whole foods and your children eat well, they are most likely getting the nutrients they need to ensure proper growth and development. In cases of a known deficiency or possibility of deficiency, you may want to take a look at making some changes to their diet or consider supplementation. But remember that all vitamins are not equal! It's important to be aware that the majority of supplements available today are synthetic. If you do choose to give your child a multivitamin, choose *food-based* supplements that can be absorbed and utilized by the body in a much more effective way than non-whole food nutrients.

Taking probiotics is another popular trend and a fairly recent practice. It is very interesting to note that people go out of their way to use 99.99

percent bacteria- and virus-killing wipes, sanitizers, soaps, and counter-top cleansers and then pay for probiotic supplements with the hopes of enhancing the bacterial flora inside their bodies! Emerging knowledge and science confirm the microbiome controls the majority of our mind-body functions and does in fact relate to many aspects of your health. What you can conclude from that is there has been sufficient microbiota within your body from the time of birth that can be supported by a natural diet and lifestyle. Ayurveda's perspective is that a person who lives in accordance with the principles of nature and follows a healthy, balanced diet and life-style that includes body and mind care has the ability to sustain healthy digestion and a balanced microbiome without the need for supplements.

RAW JUICING FOR CHILDREN

Have you ever wondered if you can offer your child a few ounces of the raw green juice you prepared at home or picked up from your local juice bar? The key concept to keep in mind is that anything raw or uncooked will be much heavier for your child's gut to digest.

As we've discussed, digestion is equivalent to cooking; the raw mate-rials broken down during the cooking process make it easy for the gut to further digest and absorb nutrients. Raw food items like raw juice have to be broken down from start to finish by the gut alone. Children with a strong digestive fire (agni) can enjoy small quantities of raw green juice without overloading their digestive system, but this should be avoided anytime you notice signs of weak digestion. There are no restrictions for fruits or fruit juices as almost all fruit is used in a ripened stage, which is nature's equivalent to cooking.

Ayurveda's principles of food and nutrition can help you support your children's body systems in growing and developing while maintaining the input of food in a seamless way, without any stagnation or deple-tion. Such a balanced flow in alignment with the principles of nature can sustain a healthy, harmonious, peaceful, and long life. Please continue to explore the inspiring world of Ayurvedic eating with your children and loved ones at home. In the next chapter, we will discover the impor-tance of water and the ways this second input can facilitate the balanced dynamics of life.

5

WATER

IT'S EASY TO see the different ways healthy food choices can support your child's overall well-being according to Ayurvedic nutrition principles, but did you know there is also a correct way to drink water? It may come as a surprise for some parents to learn that your child's daily water requirements cover more than a fixed amount of fluid or simple age-to-ounces ratio. Ayurveda still makes it easy to follow some basic guidelines without too much calculating!

First, take a moment to consider Ayurveda's concept of humans as a microcosm of the universe at large as it relates to the essential element of water—the second of the four inputs. Roughly 70 percent of both the Earth's surface and the human body consist of water, the sustenance of life necessary for the flow of all material energy. It should come as no surprise then that when it comes to water consumption and your child's health, hydration is just the tip of the iceberg. The proper regulation of this flow within the human body supports the integrity of every physiological function from a cellular level right through the final processes of elimination and purification. This includes saliva production; body temperature regulation; protection of the body's tissues, joints, and spinal cord; and creation and excretion of urine, sweat, and bowel movements—which in turn prevent constipation and urinary inflammation caused by increased concentrations of urine and acidity. Your child's water intake also helps dissolve minerals and other nutrients and facilitates optimal absorption and nutrition. Staying hydrated is just as important for your child's mental health as it is for physical health and helps the brain remain alert, focused, and attentive while maintaining cellular and chemical activities that regulate anxiety and stress levels.

Agni: The Digestive Fire

To fully appreciate the vital role water plays when it comes to your child's health, let's first explore the concept of *agni*, one of Ayurveda's core principles alongside the doshas. You might recognize this Sanskrit term meaning "fire" from earlier discussions. According to Ayurveda, agni represents the digestive fire that burns within every human being and embodies the source of life itself. Agni facilitates every stage of digestion, transformation, and metabolism and replenishes the body's tissues continuously from the time of conception until death.

Have you ever heard the expression "having a fire in your belly," often used to characterize someone as passionate or determined? In balance, agni supports a long, robust life and reflects vitality, energy, strength, radiance, a clear mind, and even lustrous skin. Out of balance—just like the doshas—it causes disease. Let's take a look at how agni works on a functional level so you can see the key role the digestive fire plays in supporting your child's optimal growth and development.

As mentioned, agni governs all the various components of digestion and metabolism and directly transforms food into nutrients. Once food is digested in the gut, agni's power of transformation continues through the entire digestive process: nutrients are absorbed and utilized by the body's various organs and tissue systems, converted into energy, and finally, the waste produced throughout the entire process of digestion and metabolism is eliminated through bowel movements, urine, and sweat. As you learned from the previous section on Ayurvedic nutrition, eating the right foods alone isn't enough if your body can't digest them.

For example, weak agni may present as low weight gain despite the fact that a child is eating plenty of food, or even consuming more food than siblings. When a child's agni is weak, Ayurveda recognizes two types of gut responses. The most common is when the child's gut identifies food as a crisis and responds with symptoms of diarrhea, stomach cramps, or vomiting. The second triggers the gut to prematurely start moving food downward, resulting in incomplete processing at each stage of digestion. Let's explore the ways weak agni impedes the normal digestive process.

Structures in the gut called sphincter muscles hold food in specific areas until the digestive process in that location is complete. The pyloric sphincter at the end of the stomach only allows its contents to move to the small intestine after pH levels indicate complete transformation. The process then continues as food passes through the ileocecal valve at the end of the small intestine into the colon. When these sphincters allow food to move to the next segment of the gut prior to completing a stage of digestion, the food your child eats can't be digested and absorbed. This manifests as poor weight gain, undernourishment, and failure to thrive. Ayurveda calls this common childhood disorder *grahani*, and it stems from low agni. Strengthening your child's agni will reinstate the disordered functions of the sphincters and is the only way to treat this condition. The advanced stage of grahani is comparable to the modern diagnosis of kwashiorkor, expressed as extreme undernourishment prevalent in many developing countries.

When your child's internal fire burns bright, absorption and assimilation of foods take place seamlessly. Digestion is strong, the doshas are nourished, and gut health improves. This in turn enhances the microbiome and supports the gut-brain axis that links the central nervous system to your stomach and intestines.

o o o

When you consider the intimate connection between the gut and brain, you can better understand the interplay between aggravated doshas, emotions, and corresponding dosha-related organs.

For example, Ayurveda considers the liver the seat of pitta. As we have discussed, excess pitta can evoke emotions such as anger and irritability. When a pitta imbalance is left uncorrected and continues to accumulate, the emotions associated with that dosha can lodge in the liver and over time even affect liver function.

o o o

On the other hand, when agni is low or weak, digestion becomes fragmented and inefficient and causes toxins known as *ama*, or undigested food, to collect in the body. Not only does accumulated ama lead to poor digestion and toxicity, but it also hinders the body's cellular intelligence and natural flow of the doshas, causing further imbalance and disease. This is the time to reignite the fire! The charts below can help you determine the strength of your child's agni and uncover possible causes of a weak digestive fire.

Signs of Various States of Agni

Status of Agni	Effect
Normal agni	Will help to properly digest food eaten in the right quantity at the right time. Promotes balanced nourishment.
Low agni	Takes a prolonged time to digest food and/or does not digest food even when taken in a moderate quantity. Tissue nourishment can be of poor quality due to malabsorption.
Fluctuating agni	Will show variability: digestion is sometimes weak, sometimes strong. This state of agni also causes variability in tissue nourishment.
Intense agni	Will digest food quickly even when taken frequently or in large quantities. If food consumption is low in quantity, it irritates the digestive tract and causes gastritis. This state of agni can cause drastic weight loss.

Common Causes and Signs of Low Agni

Causes of Low Agni	Signs of Low Agni
Eating excessively	Feeling heavy
Eating often, snacking, or eating before the previous meal is digested	Lethargy
	Dull mind
Drinking ice-cold water	Gas formation
Eating heavy, cold and/or dry foods	Constipation
Irregular eating	Bad taste in mouth
Excessive fasting. Normally, agni also gets nourished by the food we eat. In prolonged fasting, agni gets depleted, due to not getting replenished.	White-coated tongue
	Excessive saliva in mouth
	Fatigue, feeling sluggish

At the end of this chapter, you will find simple Ayurvedic recipes you can make at home to reset and strengthen your child's agni. Follow these tips to rekindle and enhance your child's digestive fire:

- Avoid overeating and/or eating heavy foods in large quantities.
- Avoid leftovers, processed food, canned foods, fast food, or food with additives and artificial coloring.
- Avoid ice water and other drinks and cold foods.
- Eat heavy foods in smaller quantities.
- Calm the mind before eating.
- Avoid prolonged fasting.
- Eat meals at regular times and avoid skipping meals without any reason.
- Drink warm water throughout the day.
- Physical exercise enhances digestion.

Remedies to Aid Digestion

These recipes are sweet with a hot and spicy taste. For children who are not accustomed to spices, you may have to add more honey. According to

Ayurveda, the subtle composition of honey undergoes chemical changes when heated, causing a reduction of its natural therapeutic properties and value that can lead to increased mucus and stagnation instead of clearing the body channels. When in doubt, use Dr. J's pinkie test: if your pinkie can comfortably tolerate the temperature, it's safe to add honey!

GINGER, SALT, AND HONEY REMEDY
Prep time: 10 minutes
INGREDIENTS
¼ teaspoon fresh ginger juice (use a grater or garlic press in
    place of a juicer) or dried ginger powder
1 teaspoon honey
Pinch of Himalayan pink salt

Mix the fresh ginger juice or dried ginger powder with the honey and a touch of Himalayan pink salt. Offer your child ½ teaspoon of this mixture 2 to 3 times a day.

CCF TEA
Prep time: 10 minutes
INGREDIENTS
½ teaspoon crushed cumin seeds
½ teaspoon crushed coriander seeds
½ teaspoon crushed fennel seeds
2 cups water
Raw honey and lemon juice to taste (optional)

This commonly used traditional Ayurvedic tea enhances digestion without overheating the body system. Boil the crushed cumin seeds, coriander seeds, and fennel seeds in the water for 5 minutes. Allow to cool to room temperature, strain, and have your child sip throughout the day. If your child is reluctant to drink because of the spicy flavor, add raw honey and freshly squeezed lemon to enhance the taste.

CORIANDER SEED TEA

Prep time: 10 minutes

INGREDIENTS

1 tablespoon crushed coriander seeds

2 cups water

Boil the crushed coriander seeds in the water for 5 minutes, then strain and cool to lukewarm for your child to sip throughout the day. This recipe is especially beneficial for children with hyperacidity and for those who cannot tolerate hot spices.

Fire and Water

You may be wondering now what this belly fire has to do with your child's water intake. Ayurveda sets forth specific principles that define how much water to drink, when to drink it, and in what form water should be consumed to maintain a healthy balance between the fire and water elements within the body. Ayurveda explains this delicate relationship in terms of opposites. Simply put: water represents cooling, heavy, and dull qualities that can dampen and smother the heat of the digestive fire when consumed improperly.

Imagine your child has a campfire in their belly. You need some kindling to get it started, but if you throw on too much, the fire will die and need to be reignited. Too much water will smother the flames. When you tend to the natural rhythms of your child's agni, you help fuel the digestive process. Following a regular eating schedule supports the body's natural intelligence in developing functional rhythms and producing digestive secretions. The best way you can support the cycle of digestion, absorption, and assimilation and ensure the food your child consumes is properly "cooked" by agni within their body is by establishing regular mealtimes.

Now that we've covered different routines to support agni, let's take a look at a couple of ways you could unknowingly be smothering the flames of your child's digestive fire and some tips to refresh the whole family's hydration habits.

Do you ever find yourself pushing your children day after day to drink more water or trying to make up for inadequate hydration in the hours after school or before bedtime? Not only is gulping down large quantities of water at one time not the best way for your kids to hydrate, it also extinguishes agni and sets the table for digestive problems at your child's next meal.

Let's see what happens to the digestive process when it's watered down to better understand the different ways water consumption can impact your child's metabolic fire. Excess fluids smother the digestive fire and dilute all the components of agni, which include saliva, stomach acids and enzymes, and bile. These diluted components then become less functional and inhibit the normal rate and process of digestion. When agni flickers, it becomes impossible for food to "cook" evenly, the same as it would if you were trying to make a meal over hot embers instead of a flame. This results in incomplete digestive transformation and poorly assimilated food that can result in a lack of nourishment and energy.

According to Ayurvedic science, the ideal ratio of food to fluids at mealtime is as follows: fill one half of the stomach with solid food, one quarter with fluids, and leave one quarter vacant for easy movement and assimilation of food in the gut. Drinking too much fluid with a meal throws off this balance and weakens digestive strength. It is interesting to note that drinking a lot of fluids at the beginning of a meal can result in weight loss and a lack of nourishment whereas drinking large amounts of fluids at the end of a meal can cause weight gain. The ideal way of hydrating at mealtimes is to sip as you eat.

Ayurveda recommends consuming larger amounts of water first thing in the morning, the only time of day the impact on agni won't interfere with digestion as your stomach is completely empty. This in turn facilitates easier bowel movements and creates more urine to flush the toxins and water from all the body systems. It's best to wait about an hour after increased water intake to have your first meal of the day so the fluid won't hamper the absorption of your breakfast.

If you aren't sure how eager your children will be to dive into a mug of water before breakfast, invite them into the kitchen with you to prepare their own kid-friendly herbal tea blends—a creative way to build this morning practice into your whole family's routine. Start out with mild flavors your children might already be familiar with like peppermint, spearmint, lemon balm, or basil. Not only will this jump-start their day, it's also the perfect way to delight your child's senses with the enticing aromas of the amazing world of herbs—a great way to introduce your kids to gardening!

Ice

If you're in the habit of dropping ice cubes into your child's beverages, it's time to rethink that next trip to the freezer! One of the most common sources of weak agni stems from drinking water at the wrong temperature—a pitfall you can easily avoid. One of the most effective ways you can set your children up for a lifetime of strong digestion and good health is to follow Ayurveda's simple recommendation to consume water either warm or at room temperature. And the same goes for you! Modifying your own lifestyle habits alongside your child's is a great way to reestablish the balance within your own body—and set an example for your kids at the same time.

You may have discovered by now that the key principles of Ayurveda remain consistent across different applications in daily life—and are actually quite intuitive. The same way you know you can douse a fire with a bucket of water, you can also weaken agni with cold beverages or ice—the quickest way to freeze digestion in its tracks. One of the greatest challenges of an Ayurvedic doctor is to convey this concept to individuals that see no problem with consuming cold or icy beverages or consistently offering them to their children. Physics is helpful to get the point across. Science is clear that cold always causes constriction and warmth always causes dilation. When you drink chilled or icy beverages, the exposure to cold causes constriction of the digestive, respiratory, circulatory, and elimination channels and leads to stagnation. Stagnation then constricts the channels of the body, slows digestive secretions, and causes feelings of heaviness in the stomach. The constriction of the respiratory channels affects oxygen intake, which in turn slows down metabolism and causes reduced energy release. Constriction also effects elimination channels and leaves bowel, urine, and sweat excretions partial, causing further dullness and lethargy. Over time, excessive cold intake can cause obesity, diabetes, high cholesterol, respiratory disorders, and diminish your child's overall health and vitality.

So in addition to hindering the digestive process in your child's belly, cold water intake also slows down metabolism. The same way swimming in a chilly pool for long periods of time can lower your child's core body temperature, so can drinking icy cold water. As the body struggles to regain its set point of 98.6 degrees (or your typical base temperature between 97 and 99 degrees), energy reserved for other processes gets rechanneled to regulate body temperature, and metabolic function slows. There is a concept in Ayurveda that the body fears exposure to cold and has a mechanism to preserve warmth as the essential aspect of our existence.

The very best way to keep children hydrated is to simply encourage them to drink small quantities of warm water by sipping throughout the day. A great tip for school-age children is to top off their water bottles before they leave for the day with some hot water left over from your morning kettle. Chances are, they won't notice the slight temperature change, and it will keep them nourished all day long. Want to make hydration more fun without adding unhealthy artificial ingredients? Encourage your kids to dive into hydration with a transparent water bottle to which you can add their favorite fresh fruit or lemon slices. This will naturally infuse the water with flavor and bring a smile to their faces!

Now that we have covered when to consume water, how to consume water, and some everyday tips on simple ways to begin new habits, let's discuss how you can best determine your child's daily water requirements according to the principles of Ayurveda.

Daily Water Requirements

Wouldn't it be nice if you could rely on your children's thirst alone as a guide to how much water they should consume? Very often, by the time kids feel the need to quench their thirst, they are already depleted or headed toward dehydration—which most parents can attest often leads to chugging copious amounts of liquids followed by a stomachache.

Ayurveda assesses daily water requirements for children based on many factors including age, constitution, activity level, and exposures to the external environment. As your child grows, their fluid intake should increase along with body weight and size, but keep in mind there is not a fixed amount of water children *should* drink based on age or any other one factor. Ayurveda offers insight into hydration based on what suits children individually and what will maintain the balance of their unique constitution.

For example, a vata child may require more fluids because the energy of vata is dry in nature. These children are generally prone to conditions including dry skin and mouth, cracked lips, and dehydration. In the case of a fiery pitta child, water requirements tend to be comparatively higher than vata as the body naturally expresses heat, causing excessive perspiration especially when pitta rises—in summertime, for example. Kapha children often require less water given the built-in nature of their constitution to retain and hold more moisture within the body system.

After you've considered your child's dosha, you'll want to look at seasons, daily weather and temperatures, and activity levels to signal your child's hydration needs. A leisurely stroll along a breezy stretch of coastline for a vata child naturally very sensitive to moving air could require the same increase in fluids as an arid desert hike on the same summer's day for a pitta child. In general, any activity or season that increases sweating requires a higher water intake, but you always want to keep your child's constitution at the helm of daily routines to prevent imbalances.

How do you know if your child is drinking enough water if you're not counting ounces? The color of your children's urine will indicate general hydration levels. When urine appears straw-colored or colorless, that means internal fluids are at an adequate level, and you should maintain your child's water intake. But anytime urine appears a deep or dark yellow, their system is becoming unbalanced, and fluids should be increased. Another useful way to assess your child's hydration status is to simply watch for signs of increased dryness throughout the body system, especially in the lips, eyes, and hands. Even when children are thirsty or dehydrated, they often forget to drink water if they are engaged with friends, games, and special projects. It can be helpful to gauge how much water your child is drinking based on the periods before lunch and then dinner in the evening. Ayurveda provides simple guidelines that can help you prevent and manage dehydration; refer to chapter 16 for more information.

Parents often wonder how much other fluid consumption over the course of a day will count toward children's overall daily water intake. After all, getting kids to drink water on its own can be a struggle, especially with the growing number of exciting, flavored hydration beverages, seltzers, and vitamin drinks available. While it isn't necessary to limit your children to a plain glass of water every time they're thirsty, be wary of sugary and artificially flavored alternatives. Do you have a child who loves seltzer water or sparkling, fizzy drinks? It is important for parents to note these beverages do not offer the same hydration benefits as plain water and are acidic in nature. Carbon dioxide (CO_2) dissolved in water is carbonic acid, which like any other acid increases tendencies to develop gastritis, GERD, feelings of burning in the stomach, and even vomiting. Feel free to offer your children fresh fruit juices and warm, organic whole milk as other healthy options alongside water—just, again, be sure they are not chilled.

This brings us to one last note on the popular trend of giving children cold smoothies blended with frozen fruit, cold milk, and various protein powders for a quick and healthy breakfast. According to Ayurvedic principles, this works directly against supporting your child's growth and development. There are a couple of reasons for this. The first consideration is the impact of cold beverages on your child's health, as we have just discussed. The second issue is incompatible food combining, as covered in chapter 4. According to Ayurveda, milk and fruit should never be consumed together; this is considered one of the worst incompatible food combinations for the digestive system. Moreover, protein powders are simply too heavy for a child's gut to digest and assimilate—it is equivalent to eating raw lentils and can cause gas formation, bloating, flatulence, and continuous burping. A much better alternative is to blend fresh fruit—not frozen—with previously boiled nondairy oat or rice milk, or almond milk with some dry roasted nuts (which are easily digestible), and a touch of a refreshing spice like cardamom.

As we have explored, water is an essential component to maintain balanced nutrition, circulation, immunity, and elimination. Too little water or too much water causes turbulence in our physiology and leads to imbalances. A personalized approach to children's hydration habits is another Ayurvedic routine to help maintain day-to-day health. A balanced flow of the four inputs through our body in alignment with the flow of nature helps achieve sustainable health and longevity. Now, we will turn our attention to the third input: the breath—the flow of prana through our body that sustains life.

6

BREATH

HOW MANY TIMES have you found yourself eye level with your child in the midst of a meltdown telling them to take a deep breath when they are upset or frustrated? If you're like most parents, chances are high that one of the first ways you encourage your children to calm down when they're distressed about something is by focusing on their breath. You might even wonder why it can be so difficult for your children to regain composure and get themselves back on track. After all, everyone knows how to breathe. So why is this so much easier said than done?

Just Breathe

While it's simple to instruct your children to calm down and relax, if they don't have more specific and effective tools to diminish negative feelings and restore inner calm, they really have no way of managing big emotions. In those moments when they feel overwhelmed and out of control, your stepping in and soothing them makes all the difference. Asking them over and over to do the impossible on their own can often make them even more frustrated and upset—as you may have experienced yourself at times. In the same way you would never expect a child to know how to tie their shoes or ride a bicycle without instruction and practice, you can't expect children to know how they can calm themselves down using deep breaths unless you first teach them how to breathe.

According to Ayurveda and yoga, the breath is a direct channel to the mind. Different patterns of breathing create distinct effects and energies that can be either stimulating or stabilizing, heating or cooling, or uplifting or grounding. When you customize breathing rhythms in combination with lifestyle routines based on your child's unique constitution and state of health, you can achieve immediate and sustainable outcomes.

All it takes to guide your children through simple, fun breathing exercises is a few minutes a day—and the benefits to their lives will be many—including emotional and self-regulation, enhanced focus and concentration, increased learning ability, decreased stress and anxiety, and a balanced and joyful state of being. Recent studies recognize the beneficial effects of mindfulness tools on the well-being of children and adolescents, and the importance of these techniques specifically as a protocol for managing learning disabilities, sensory processing disorders, and autism. One such study conducted by the head of Brain and Neurocognitive Development at Ural Federal University and published in the journal *Biological Psychiatry* studied the effects of diaphragmatic rhythmic deep breathing, or belly breathing, on children with ADHD. The research showed that yoga and breathing exercises improve attention, decrease hyperactivity, and help children to engage in complex activities for longer periods of time. Concentrated breathwork supplies the brain with more oxygen, which in turn helps the part of the brain responsible for regulation of brain activity known as reticular formation—deficient in children with ADHD—and begins to regulate a child's state of activity.[1]

If making room on your priority list for mindfulness exercises amid the chaos of a busy schedule seems challenging, think of it as being as essential for your child as getting fresh air and physical exercise or eating healthy foods. According to Ayurveda, one of the most important ways you can nurture your child's mind and body is by making time to practice different breathing techniques together. When you adopt simple mindfulness routines in your everyday life, you promote feelings of well-being and happiness in your children and bring your whole family together in the present moment—something parents today long for more than ever in a culture of increased disconnection.

While "Just breathe" has taken off as a popular mantra lately, breath-work as a root principle of Ayurveda extends back thousands of years and can become one of the most powerful and effective tools in your parenting kit.

Pranayama

What if I told you there was a way to seamlessly sync your children's mind and body—much like you do with your digital devices—that could guide them along a path to stay healthy and balanced throughout their lives? Both the Ayurvedic system of medicine and yoga recognize the breath as the vital essence of life. You can, in fact, visualize the breath as the bridge that connects the mind and body.

It's easy to see the different variations of breathing patterns that occur with physical activity and different emotions or states of mind. Targeted breathwork applies the same principles to influence the body and mind and achieve specific outcomes by implementing controlled techniques and pacing of the breath.

Pranayama, or the art of breathing, literally means "regulation of breath" or "control over the breath." Beyond its vital role of providing oxygen, energy, and sustaining life, the breath regulates the physiological and psychological functions of the body and harmonizes the mind-body connection. As you may have come across yourself in your own research on breathing or meditation, pranayama has noted and measurable positive effects on brain function and mental activity. When you regulate or streamline breathing patterns, you can achieve specific outcomes and make the necessary mental and physical shifts to bring the body into a state of overall balance.

Maybe you've heard the term in a yoga class before or felt the effects of pranayama yourself at times you've simply brought attention to your breath when taking a deep inhalation or exhaling a long, audible sigh of relief, for example. It's easy to see the different ways breathing with awareness can recalibrate your emotions and mental activity at any moment and how your children can use this essential tool in their every-day life to do the same.

Prana—one of the eight limbs of yoga—is a subtle form of energy carried through the breath that governs the interplay between mind and body. Have you ever noticed that your breath becomes shallow, rapid, and irregular when you feel nervous or upset? Or that it turns slower and rhythmic when you're content or happily absorbed in a book or project? In the same way thought patterns affect the quality of your breath, different pranayama techniques or rhythms of breathing can facilitate different perceptions, thoughts, and feelings.

Overall, the process of inhalation and exhalation has four distinct steps. The first is to fill the lungs. Then, after breathing in there is an undefined, unregulated pause when the lungs completely expand. Next comes the purifying exhalation that eliminates carbon dioxide, or impure breath. Finally, another undefined, unregulated pause follows the exhalation before the cycle continues. The practice of pranayama regulates the duration of these four different stages of the cycle and allows you to experience definite emotional and physiological changes—an invaluable tool you can offer your children to connect the mind and body.

BELLY BREATHING

While it may seem next to impossible for you to imagine the ways you might help your children regulate their breath when some days feel like a never-ending struggle to regulate their behavior, the truth is it's easier than you think. With just a few tips you can equip your kids with simple breathing techniques and successfully help them along anyplace, anytime. The key is to teach them in a fun, encouraging way—and to join in yourself, of course! The benefits of pranayama aren't just for your children.

Do you ever wonder how it's possible your child can have so much energy at the very moment it's time to climb into bed when they've spent the entire day running around and burning off energy? Parents frequently find bedtime challenging for children—a time of day when it can be hard for them to wind down and relax and for parents to say goodnight and enjoy some personal time. As most parents can attest to, children of all ages frequently have bedtime worries and often resist turning the light off with a stream of creative excuses designed to avoid going to sleep. One of the best breathing exercises you can practice with your child to ease nighttime anxieties and prepare the mind-body system for rest is deep breathing or belly breathing. You can incorporate this calming exercise into your child's bedtime routine nightly, just like bathing or brushing their teeth. Doing so will habituate your child's mind and body to the practice and automatically signal their system to go to sleep after just a few deep breaths.

Belly breathing, also known as diaphragmatic breathing, is a simple pranayama technique perfect to share with your children at bedtime that regulates the breath cycle with deep inhalations followed by long exhalations. Ask your child to do a simple experiment and place their hand on their belly: when they breathe in does their belly expand? You'd be surprised how many kids and adults breathe all wrong, completely the other way around! Make corrections as needed and ask your child to be mindful that taking deep breaths helps them feel better. Discuss the importance of breathing in as energizing and nourishing and breathing out as relaxing and a time to wish the day farewell.

Once your child is cozy in bed, ask them to lie on their back and place a hand, stuffed animal, or even a favorite small object on their belly. Guide them to inhale deeply through their nose into their belly and watch the object move upward, then slowly breathe out through their mouth and notice their abdomen move downward. Have your child focus their attention on this rising and falling belly ten to fifteen times or until you sense they feel relaxed and ready for a peaceful night's sleep.

You can use this same technique whenever children feel angry or irritated. One of the best ways to reduce negative emotions and restore a feeling of calm to children's minds is to hold them close and ask them to take deep inhalations followed by long exhalations. After a couple of minutes, they will feel more content and come back to the present moment. Over time, children will connect to the stillness and peace of their body's relaxation response and have the ability to continue this breathing exercise on their own when they feel anxious or restless.

Perhaps there are other times during the day when your family might benefit from slowing down and taking a few deep breaths together. Is there a particular weeknight jam-packed with scheduled commitments or periods of time spent in the car that you could use to focus on a short breathing exercise? Many parents find this a wonderful and easy morning ritual to practice with their children before school, for example—a time to boost feelings of calm and help them stay focused and relaxed all day long in the classroom.

Ayurveda offers many practical suggestions you can apply in your daily life that will nurture the seeds of mindfulness within your children and help create a happier and more peaceful life. We will discuss more specific breathing techniques you can practice according to your child's dosha later in this chapter.

The Mindful Child

Most parents do everything they can to raise kindhearted and loving children, but many have never encountered the link between mindfulness and compassion. Ayurveda clearly conveys that a mindful child is one who is able to perceive everything around them in a stable, balanced way and respond in kind to their environment and peers. When you practice simple mindfulness techniques with your children, you teach them how to be fully in touch with feelings of joy and peace that support a bright, clear perspective along with learning, creativity, and connection to friends, peers, and community.

Would it surprise you to know that children who regularly practice deep breathing exercises or even just naturally take a lot of deep breaths are generally calmer and better able to focus on different learning assignments or hobbies in an especially easy way? Mindful children enjoy clear perception in the same way a calm lake flawlessly reflects its surroundings, undisturbed by ripples or distortion. We will look more deeply at perception when we discuss different qualities of the child's mind and effects of sensory inputs in the next chapter.

When you show your children different ways to practice mindfulness by simply taking time with them each day to breathe deeply or connect with the beauty of nature, for example, you help them learn to be compassionate not only with others, but so importantly, with themselves.

Simple and focused attention on the present moment teaches children at an early age how to build self-esteem, take care of negative emotions, and be less overwhelmed by strong feelings.

Children who practice breathing techniques and have learned how to breathe deeply and keep their breath steady not only see things more clearly but also remain less affected by sudden emotional stimuli. Think about a classroom—an environment where children can easily become overwhelmed or anxious when a teacher reprimands another student for misbehaving or disrupting the class, as an example. Children often internalize these negative emotions and experiences and connect themselves to what is going on around them externally. A child who has cultivated mindfulness, on the other hand, can clearly perceive the situation exists between the misbehaving classmate and teacher and will be able to separate themselves from the negative stimuli. In this way, simple breathing practices can help children learn to observe strong emotions and changes in their environment without allowing those changes to affect them or take root in negative ways.

Despite every parent's wish to protect their children from pain or distress of any kind, it's inevitable that your child will face many different circumstances in their day-to-day life—some pleasant and some not so pleasant. Your job as a conscious parent is to help your child cultivate an ability to face life's unpredictable situations as a witness and not be consumed by the stressors and changes of their environment. Ayurveda clearly conveys that stress is not measured by what is happening in the outside world, but by the ways your mind and body are altered by them. Pranayama is a powerful tool that can empower children to witness changes in their external environment while remaining calm and separate.

Parenthood affords many opportunities to invite mindfulness into your child's life and being in nature is a great place to start. Nature brings out the nurturing and curious qualities in children in a myriad of ways while hiking through the woods, for example, or surrounded by blue sky and the wonderful sounds of life. Not only do children feel an enhanced sense of peace and grounding being outside, but they seamlessly connect to metaphors found in the natural world. Introduce your child to the following mindfulness practice on your next walk outside along with a breathing exercise to practice at home or anywhere your child experiences negative emotions.

CLOUD BREATH

Have you ever stopped with your child on a windy day to observe the clouds moving across the sky? Explain to your child how clouds are like their emotions that simply travel through their body the same way clouds travel through the sky. Soon, they will float away and be gone. In the same way children understand the weather outside is not permanent and is always changing, they can easily understand stormy weather inside of them as clouds merely passing by. When it's raining outside, or even thundering and lightning, children wait calmly for the sun to come out again. They know the storm will not last forever. You can help your children understand their emotions the same way; a temporary weather condition passing through the sky.

When you're ready to guide them through a breathing practice, first ask them to visualize a great big, blue sky. Next, ask them to choose a cloud on which they'd like to place a thought or feeling that would then float away. Your child can either visualize that feeling outside of them sailing away on a cloud or can use long exhalations from the deep breathing exercise to slowly help the cloud move through the sky until it drifts away.

Depending on your family's interests and hobbies, you may or may not spend a lot of time in nature on a regular basis. When you take time outside with your children, it encourages them to observe the flow of nature itself and helps develop mindfulness. It could be something as simple as watching a bee move from flower to flower sucking up nectar from different plants or a mother crow feeding and caring for her young. Nature is the best teacher and the best healer. Even just standing barefoot on the earth or hugging a tree with your forehead resting on the trunk can instantly relieve stress headaches and tension. The same way Mother Nature supports a plant from seed to sprout to bloom, the Earth can also absorb our imbalances and energize and nurture the entire mind-body system. Connecting to the Earth in any form releases aggravated energy and offers a deeply grounding experience for your children.

Breathing Techniques for the Doshas

Children's energy levels can swing from day to day and even change by the hour, just like yours. Have you ever noticed how some days your children are bouncing off the walls and on others they can barely get off the couch? You can follow these cues along with a child's Ayurvedic constitution to identify current imbalances and help bring the doshas back into equilibrium. The following pranayama techniques can be tailored to your child's dosha or a reflection of a predominant imbalance—another tool to incorporate into your child's daily routines to support health, vitality, and balance. While breathing techniques are a simple practice you can explore at home with your children, it is ideal to consult a qualified yoga practitioner or Ayurvedic professional to instruct and customize breathwork for your child. Elaborate and prolonged pranayama practices are primarily suggested for adults, but even a minute or two of simple breathing practices as a fun activity with your children can help them experience the benefits of these techniques and introduce them to the practice.

VATA

Are there times your child has difficulty focusing or a tendency to be restless and easily distracted? As you probably recognize, these are expressions of vata dosha or of a vata imbalance. One of the simplest and most effective breathing techniques to pacify vata is Alternate Nostril Breathing, or *Nadi Shodhana*, in ancient texts, meaning "clearing the channels."

Invite your child to sit cross-legged on the floor next to you with a tall spine and show them how to close their right nostril with their right thumb and use belly breathing to inhale through their left nostril. Then show them how to switch fingers and close the left nostril with their right ring finger and exhale through their right nostril. Repeat these steps while alternating nostrils and breathing slowly and easily, without any force. You will find that even practicing this breath for one to two minutes every day with your child can increase feelings of calm, stability, and focus for you both. Alternate Nostril Breathing is one of the simplest breathing techniques you can practice and is known for calming the nervous system, reducing stress and anxiety, balancing hormones, promoting clarity of mind and concentration, and improving neuromuscular coordination, blood circulation, and cardiovascular health. This is breathwork that balances both sides of the brain, can be done sitting or lying down, and has no contraindications. It is very powerful and effective for reducing anxiety and stress and balancing the body and the sympathetic and parasympathetic nervous systems.

PITTA

Do you have children who are hotheaded or quickly irritated by nature? Challenge your children to these next stabilizing breathing exercises anytime you notice a fiery pitta predominance that needs cooling off—a go-to breathing technique in summertime!

This next breath in Ayurveda and yoga is called Sheetali, which means "cooling," and is also referred to sometimes as Seetkari, meaning "performed with a hissing sound." First, find a cool place to sit and ask your child to clench their teeth with their tongue resting inside their mouth while they open their lips the same way they would when brushing their teeth. Encourage them to try and breathe through their mouth by sucking the air in through the space between their teeth with a hissing sound then exhaling slowly through their nose. Continue a few times before relaxing together.

Another method of performing this cooling breath is to keep the tongue out and folded in the shape of a straw or tube. Breathe in slowly through the mouth into the tube and notice the cool feeling of the air against the mouth, throat, and palate. Once the inhalation is complete, close the mouth and exhale through the nose. These cooling breathing practices not only pacify pitta and decrease body heat but also support liver and skin health and reduce acidity, excessive sweating, and feelings of anger, frustration, and agitation of the mind.

KAPHA

Sometimes children require a more invigorating breath to stimulate energy levels and get them moving. Do you notice your child acting especially lazy or procrastinating more than usual when it comes to homework or chores, for example? A kapha-type child will move at a slower pace by nature compared to other children, but any increase in slowness or lack of motivation may signal an imbalance. This playful, brightening breath known as *Kapalabhati*, or the Breath of Fire, will lighten and energize your child's entire mind-body system. Breath of Fire enhances metabolism, boosts cognition, improves circulation, supports weight management, purifies the nervous system, and reduces anxiety and depression.

Invite your child to sit in a comfortable position on the floor next to you with a tall spine and show them how to inhale passively then exhale forcefully through the nose while contracting your abdominal muscles without strain. Demonstrate a couple cycles of this breath, then practice a few rounds together and ask them to stay relaxed and notice the enhanced circulation and energy flow throughout their body. Kapalabhati is often recommended for children who are diabetic but contraindicated for kids with hyperacidity. Kapalabhati can be done by vata types in a slow rhythmic fashion, should be avoided by pitta types or performed with prolonged exhalation to avoid overheating, and is very useful for kapha types.

Adapting Breathwork for Your Child

Keep in mind as a general principal, vata requires calming breathwork, kapha requires stimulating exercises, and pitta needs cooling breathwork. This short list and the breathing exercises that follow can be helpful when deciding which techniques are best for your children based on their dosha.

VATA

They benefit from abdominal breathing, full yogic breathing, and Alternate Nostril Breathing. For issues with elimination, Kapalabhati done in the morning can ease constipation.

PITTA

Cooling breathwork like Sheetali pranayama followed by Alternate Nostril Breathing and Bhramari are great for pitta. Exhalations should be longer than inhalations, and smooth rhythmic breathing with brief suspension of breath after exhalation helps.

KAPHA

Kapalabhati, Bhastrika, and Surya Bhedana followed by Alternate Nostril Breathing would be great for stimulating kaphas. They benefit from rhythmic breathing and gentle exhalation retention. Ujjayi reduces kapha particularly in the throat and increases the digestive fire. Generally breathwork stimulates and increases the Air and Space elements, which counteract the Earth and Water elements in the body and reduce kapha accumulation in lungs, chest, sinuses, and stomach.

TRIDOSHA-PACIFYING BREATHWORK

Nadi Shodhana and Bhastrika are considered Tridosha pacifying; they alleviate vata issues related to the joints and nervous system, remove excess kapha from stomach and lungs to aid respiration and digestion, and address pitta issues related to digestion as well. The same Bhastrika that can aggravate pitta and make vata spacey, if done mindfully, can pacify all doshas. There are contraindications though: Bhastrika should not be done by pregnant women or people with hypertension or cardiac issues, and this knowledge is essential for all the healing practices.

Simple Breathing Exercises for Children

The key to practicing any type of breathwork with your kids is to make it fun! Join in, be silly, and keep the language you use easy to understand . . . and the breath will follow. Here are simple, fun breathing exercises you can practice anytime.

BUMBLEBEE BREATH (BHRAMARI)

Close your eyes, plug your ears, inhale through the nose, and quietly hum as you exhale. Repeat this three to five times. This soothes the nervous system, calms and focuses the mind, and is great for the vocal chords!

BUNNY BREATH

Pretend you're a bunny, take three quick inhales in through your nose, and then let out one long exhale. Repeat this three to five times. This is a great practice to manage anxiety.

THREE-PART BREATH

This breath promotes breathing deeply and expanding all parts of the lungs to refresh and supply air to the entire body. The in-breath should start in the bottom third of the body from below the navel to the base of the ribs, then you continue to fill the ribs to the heart, and pause and fill the top portion from heart to skull. While exhaling, do so from top to bottom in a smooth long exhale, squeezing the belly at the end of the exhale. Repeat from bottom to top and exhale from top to bottom.

SURYA AND CHANDRA BHEDANA PRANAYAMA

Breathing from the right nostril with the left closed is heating and called Surya Bhedana, while breathing from the left nostril with the right closed is called Chandra Bhedana. A few rounds of these can be done based on doshas and seasons but do follow them up with Alternate Nostril Breathing for balancing.

BALLOON BREATHING

While sitting or lying down, hands on your thighs or by your sides, palms facing upward, inhale and fill your body like a big balloon. Then exhale and blow the air out through your mouth. Repeat this three to five times. This can be done before sleeping for deeper rest.

OCEAN BREATH (UJJAYI)

Imagine a hot day when you take a drink of water from the fridge and sigh after that with your mouth open! Now close your mouth and make the same sound from the back of your throat, which sounds like an ocean. This is a calming breath and a few rounds at bedtime can promote sound sleep.

BELLOWS BREATH (BHASTRIKA)

Kneel down on a soft surface, such as a yoga mat or a folded towel, with toes and knees together, and sit back on your heels with spine erect. Sit up tall and relax your shoulders, then bend your elbows and make loose fists with your hands, bringing them next to your shoulders with elbows close to the body. Take a transition breath in and out. Then breathe in through the nostrils, inhaling forcefully, and raise your hands straight overhead into the air, opening up your fists and spreading fingers wide. Exhale with force through the nostrils while bringing your arms back to the starting position and making fists again with your hands. Continue inhaling as you raise your hands, then exhale for five to ten sets, pausing in between for 15–30 seconds. You can repeat this up to three times. This is an energizing breath and a great pick-me-up. It cleanses the lungs and exercises muscles. It can aggravate pitta and make vata spacey but is very helpful in reducing kapha-associated sluggishness and stagnation, especially from the head and chest.

RHYTHMIC BREATHING TO A COUNT

Breathe in to a count of four, hold to a count of two, breathe out to a count of six (a longer exhale), and hold again to a count of two. The count can vary, but this type of rhythmic breathing slows down the mind.

Before you begin your exciting pranayama journey, please give consideration to the following breathwork guidelines and be mindful that pranayama must be practiced on a consistent basis to achieve the most positive outcome for your children.

- Avoid any breathwork when feeling very hungry or immediately after a meal.
- Never hurry through breathing exercises. Choose a time that works for your family and can support your child to have a focused and mindful practice.
- Avoid any stimulating breathing exercises when your child is very anxious, worried, or angry. Opt for slow, deep breathing or cooling and stabilizing breaths at those times.
- Avoid breathwork after your child returns from physical exertion or exercise.
- Make sure your child is stable, calm, relaxed, and focused before guiding them through any breathwork.
- Avoid specific breathwork other than normal, regular breathing when your child has any type of sickness, fever, congestion, or a runny nose.

What children want most from parents is love and attention. When you take time out of your busy life to practice mindfulness techniques with your children, it shows them you are present and committed to their well-being and eager to embark on new journeys together. This fills them with great confidence and joy and helps to integrate all of the tools Ayurveda offers to harmonize the physical, mental, and emotional aspects of your child's mind-body system. It all starts with you . . . take a deep breath!

7

PERCEPTION

IF YOU STOP to think about the different ways you perceive the world around you or how your children perceive their day-to day experiences beyond what meets the eye, you'll realize the truth of the expression "perception is everything." Ayurveda considers the five senses the portals that connect your child with the external world. Not only are these perceptions the basis for what creates your child's reality, but they have tremendous influence on their physical health and well-being across all of the body systems including digestion, metabolism, immune strength, and even hormonal health.

According to Ayurveda, perception is all of the information perceived through the five senses: the ears, nose, tongue, eyes, and skin—the portals for transmitting stimuli to the mind. Imbalanced perceptions stem from abnormal use of the senses and result in distorted responses of the mind— why Ayurveda considers mind care so important. Mind care means looking after all of the senses so information and experiences can be clearly perceived and responded to in a balanced way. The four inputs (ahara) in human life are food, water, breath, and perception, and Ayurveda considers perception the most important.

The Trigunas

Have you ever wondered how two children—maybe even your own—can respond to the exact same situation in completely different ways? To understand the qualities of mind that lead to these variations, we need to explore some concepts central to Ayurveda.

According to Ayurveda, nature consists of three primordial qualities called *trigunas* that are responsible for the diversity of all existence. These three cosmic qualities are *sattva*, the primal intelligence that imparts balance; *rajas*, the energy responsible for activity or movement and intensity; and *tamas*, the heaviness that creates inertia. Every substance in the cosmos—matter, energy, mind, and life—embodies different combinations of these three qualities—just as the human system does. The qualities of the trigunas can be observed in the world around us and are also expressed both in the physical body and as attributes of the mind, governing the ways individuals perceive and respond to the world around them.

The quality of sattva represents goodness, intelligence, balance, and harmony. Sattva carries mental attributes of contentment, happiness, clarity, purity, and peace and will never causes any imbalances. Rajas is the quality of movement, activity, intensity, turbulence, and changes. Rajas brings action, competition, power, and stimulation and can lead to conflict and distress. Tamas represents darkness and qualities of inertia, heaviness, dullness, stagnation, and decay. It produces delusion, sleep, ignorance, animosity, and insensitivity.

Since rajas and tamas can cause imbalances, they are also considered the doshas of the mind—the primary reason for mental imbalances. Calmness and clarity of the mind are essential for clear, stable perception—the main attributes of sattva. Becoming more sattvic through mind care creates stability and clarity, allows you to see the truth of everything, and provides focus, devotion, and light. Tamas and rajas, on the other hand, cause mental unrest that triggers agitation, misperception, and delusion.

Management of the mind in Ayurveda and yoga are primarily directed toward enhancing sattva and minimizing rajas and tamas so that the mind can perceive things clearly and avoid delusions. All stimuli brought in through the senses will be reflected the same way they are perceived, based on the prevailing qualities of an individual's mind. A child who has a sattvic-predominant mind will have the ability to discern everything around them clearly without any distortion and respond the same way. Sattva helps us to see things clearly and assess without any exaggeration or judgment—what is commonly known as mindfulness.

Your child's mind is like a sponge, absorbing whatever comes through the portals of the five senses without any filter or differentiation between positive and negative. Everything your children perceive becomes their internal reality and a pure reflection of their exposures on the mirror within. This process is completely different for adults, as we see or hear things in reference to the collection of our previous experiences. The adult mind automatically starts differentiating the good from the bad and the positive from the negative based on past stimuli. This is why you sometimes see your child observing situations and experiences without any immediate reaction, whether it is a trip to the amusement park or a quarrel or conflict. Everything children perceive is digested within and becomes their reference point for the future.

Perception centers around the different ways your child's mind gets influenced and triggered based on what they hear, see, taste, smell, or feel every day. In fact, children can sometimes develop health problems due to their imbalanced perceptions about certain situations that even parents may find hard to unravel. Dr. J had a consultation once with a fifth grader who had developed intermittent indigestion and constipation due to fear triggered by a teacher who had reprimanded her for talking during class on her first day of school. The parent's only feedback from their child up to that point had been that the teacher was loving and caring, and they couldn't figure out what was causing their daughter's symptoms to emerge. A detailed history revealed this fear and helped explain the underlying trigger for the symptoms so they could help their daughter and seek counseling and support.

The mind is very subtle and even minor inputs can have great impacts on your child's body system. This is why Ayurveda says, "Mind care is life care." Often, the biggest challenge for parents is not being able to identify the struggles going on within their child's mind. The best way to stay connected to your children and support them through the different challenges they will face throughout every stage of childhood is by creating a space for them to feel safe and comfortable discussing things and sharing their true feelings with you. Your presence and close attention on a consistent basis are the best way to support your child's mind.

Mind Care

Your child's mind is like a blank canvas that you can assist in developing into a wonderful creation full of bright colors and vitality with the right brushstrokes. This is a wonderful opportunity for parents to enhance the vibrancy of life's experiences and allow these creations to flourish on the canvas of your child's mind by being emotionally available, guiding them in a positive way, and protecting them from negative perceptions.

There are many ways you can enhance the colors of your child's imagination and support the complete development of their mind. Children are very curious by nature and may have numerous questions every day for you, for instance—even some you may find silly or not age-appropriate. When you take the time to answer any questions that may hold a serious place in your child's mind regardless of how they are presented with patience and attention, you support your children on every level and also give them correct information so they don't seek it from another source that could be potentially harmful—another way you are protecting your child. Never ignore or suppress your children's questions, as these are a pathway to providing them noble, accurate information to help them clarify the uncertainties in their minds.

Another example of how you can take care of your child's mind is protecting your children from various exposures. Parents have different philosophies about what is best for their children when it comes to engaging with the world. There are extreme approaches on both ends of the spectrum: imposing many restrictions on children as well as allowing children to be exposed to everything and leaving them on their own to figure out how to deal with it. Neither will reinforce the proper development of your child's mind and allow them the best ability to live a healthy, positive life. Too many restrictions inhibit children's evolution as confident and independent individuals, while allowing them to do whatever they want leaves them vulnerable without any guidance or backup and can shift them into a habit of fear and insecurity. Similarly, imposing restrictions on what naturally inspires your children or forcing them to do things they don't like to do without any reason can create the negativity of anger, frustration, and sadness and sometimes develop a rebellious mentality. Let's look at ways to avoid these pitfalls.

Improper Use of the Senses

Did you know that you can support and protect the health of your child's five senses? Ayurveda identifies improper use of the senses as one of the main causes of imbalances that can lead to health problems. There are three types of improper use of senses: excessive exposure, deficient exposure, and altered exposure. Examples of these would be reading in extremely bright light, very dim light, or flickering light. The first is an excessive exposure to the eyes. Reading in a very dim light is an exposure of deficiency. And reading in flickering light is an altered, or erratic and irregular, exposure. Not only do all of these exposures cause eyestrain, they can also lead to other systemic problems—even mental disorders as you can see from the following table. Just as you can support your children's digestion by making healthy food choices and establishing regular mealtimes for them, you can also support their senses through optimal exposures. The health of your child's five senses is essential for preventing imbalances as well as for enhancing your child's individual potential.

Signs and Symptoms of Improper Use of the Senses

Sense Organ	Physical Signs and Symptoms	Mental Signs and Symptoms
Eye/Vision	Eye pain, vision issues, headache, exhaustion	Memory issues, irritability
Ear/Sound	Earache, deafness, sleep issues, dizziness, tinnitus	Stress, aggression, fear
Nose/Smell	Loss of sense of smell, pain in the nose, dryness of nose	Confusion, mental dullness
Tongue/Taste	Altered sense of taste, loss of sense of taste, indigestion, lack of nourishment	Restlessness of mind, lack of concentration
Skin/Touch	Altered sense of touch, burning skin, skin injury, skin irritation	Feeling of isolation

Parenting in the Digital Age

The inevitable sensory overload from modern life and technology is one of the most challenging issues in children's lives today. Parents are often unaware of the everyday impacts and damage this causes to their children's minds and bodies and of the simple steps they can take to minimize reactions and restore balance. Your children are exposed to computers, digital screens, tablets, and cell phones on a regular basis, which cause an excessive load on their senses and stress to their mind-body systems. Because of their young age, this can affect development and even lead to early weakness and degenerations.

In addition to the effects of media and screen time on a child's mind and body, the electromagnetic field (EMF) created by Wi-Fi, cellular networks, and other electronic appliances at home interferes with natural physiology, processes of the mind, and emotional stability. It is very common today for children to have sleep disorders, increased irritability, headaches, dizziness, and a hard time concentrating from these increasing exposures. Dr. J has seen a rise in a number of such conditions in children over the last decade. Parents should consider taking measures to reestablish balance, including minimizing exposures to EMFs by keeping devices in airplane mode while not in use, switching off the Wi-Fi modem, and moving children's bedrooms away from any electrical smart meters.

Restoring the Senses

Protecting your child from improper use of the senses is ideal, but it may seem impractical in our technology-driven modern world. In such unavoidable situations in life, the only practical approach is to focus on how we can counterbalance occurrences that lie outside of our control in the same way we manage the doshas. The best ways to support your child's five senses are to support them first and foremost in going to sleep early, taking breaks related to specific sensory exposures, and getting outside in nature multiple times a day to help their senses and mind realign from the wear and tear of the day. Getting enough sleep at night is essential for many reasons, as we will discover in the next chapter, as it is the only time the mind and senses can relax, repair, recoup, and rejuvenate. Ayurveda provides specific guidance to support the sense organs you can easily implement at home to help balance and protect your child's senses and perception, as you can see from this table.

Sense Organ	Remedies and Practices for Supporting Specific Senses
Eye/Vision	Splash water on the face, as it has a cooling and stabilizing effect on the eyes. Apply ghee on the eyelids and around the eyes.
Ear/Sound	Apply sesame oil in the ear.
Nose/Smell	Apply one drop of Anu Thailam or Nasya oil inside the nostrils with the pinkie or a Q-tip.
Tongue/Taste	Scrape the tongue in the morning with a tongue scraper after brushing the teeth. Rinse the mouth with one teaspoon of Arimedadi Thailam oil, and then spit it out.
Skin/Touch	Apply either sesame oil or a constitution-based Ayurvedic oil all over the body, keep it on for at least fifteen minutes, and then wash it off with natural soap or shampoo, ideally once a day or at least once or twice a week.

Each and every experience children have on a day-to-day basis is an opportunity for them to develop their cognitive skills, minds, imaginations, and talents. The key to ensure your child's optimal growth and development is to contribute to well-rounded, positive exposures that will in turn support your children to have balanced and clear perceptions.

PART THREE

Daily Routines, Lifestyle Tools, and Everyday Care for Your Child

8

SLEEP

WHEN WAS THE last time you got a good night's sleep? For busy parents who may be sleep-deprived themselves, this can be a tough question to answer—and may even feel like a luxury! But when it comes to your children, you probably don't take these disruptions as lightly. In fact, your child's sleep routines likely carry great significance in the quality of your day-to-day life. It's easy to see how going to bed too late, waking up too early, or missing the nap window often leads to cranky behavior and tantrums, turning sleep-deprived kids from sweet to scary in the blink of an eye.

According to Ayurveda, sleep is one of the three pillars of life essential for health and well-being. Its fundamental role within our bodies is best conveyed in direct translation from the Vedic text: "Happiness, nourishment, strength, virility, knowledge, and life itself depend on proper sleep"!

Benefits of Sleep

Establishing a regular bedtime is an important part of the Ayurvedic daily routine for all age groups to ensure health, harmony, peace, happiness, and longevity. And the benefits of healthy sleep go well beyond feeling rested, especially for children. A good night's sleep enhances learning ability, heightens focus and attention, sharpens memory, balances emotions, and improves quality of life. When your children go to bed too late or experience disturbed sleep, it can lead to many mind-body problems including fatigue, constipation, low energy, impaired mood regulation, a lack of focus, falling asleep in the classroom, and of course, increased irritability—which, as you know, can persist for an entire day. The American Academy of Pediatrics estimates that sleep problems impact 25–50 percent of children and 40 percent of adolescents. Sleep deprivation is a public health crisis in the United States and has grave mental and physical health impacts on children and adolescents that often continue right into adulthood:

- Poor sleep in early childhood has been linked to allergic rhinitis, immunity issues, obesity, diabetes, and anxiety and depression.
- It may lead to disorders of the immune system and increase susceptibility to infections.
- It has been linked to anxiety and depression.
- It can lead to attention and behavioral issues.
- It can cause future cardiovascular risks.
- It can increase the chances of developing type 2 diabetes, obesity, and high blood pressure.
- It can worsen cognitive and academic performance and mental health.
- Sleep deprivation can cause car crashes and sports injuries in teens.

Sound Sleep

Sleep is not the same as rest—and while periods of rest are important for everyone's health and well-being, they cannot make up for lost sleep. Rest on its own will not compensate for or prevent sleep deprivation because sleep is when both the body *and* the mind rest and is the time for mental digestion as well as processing of all the day's sensory impressions. As mentioned, Ayurveda considers sleep one of the three pillars of a balanced life and, for this reason, gives much more importance to the hours your child is asleep than the hours your child is awake. From the time your child wakes up in the morning until they go to sleep at night, there is constant wear and tear on the body, mind, and senses. Sleep is the prime time for recovery and recuperation and for critical physiological processes that occur during different stages of sleep such as healing tissue injuries from the day, brain waste clearance, energy preservation, modulation of immune responses, cognition, repair of brain cells, and restoration of vitality. Most importantly, though, all of the information your child gathered throughout the day through sensory perceptions and experiences of the mind, like what they learned in school that day, as an example, is reconsolidated from the frontal cortex of the brain to long-term memory. This can only occur during the deepest state of sleep.

Bedtimes for Children

Early to bed and early to rise is the Ayurvedic mantra for maintaining good health and ensuring longevity. Your children need a lot more sleep than you do, as they are in the growing phase of their life. Activity causes depletion, and sleep facilitates nourishment and growth.

According to Ayurveda, children between three and six years old need to sleep for more than half of the full twenty-four hours in a day. The required twelve or thirteen hours don't need to be in a single stretch at night but can instead be broken up into ten to eleven hours at night and one to two hours in an afternoon nap. It is ideal for children of all ages to go to bed by 8 p.m. and wake by 6 or 7 a.m. Children over the age of six need an average of ten to twelve hours of sleep a day. As you well know, the afternoon nap has either been shortened or completely given up at this age. Teenagers over thirteen need eight to ten hours of sleep. According to the CDC, six out of ten middle schoolers and seven out of ten high schoolers are not getting a sufficient amount of sleep.

The Ayurvedic daily routine is based on when you go to sleep—the time that determines when you wake up. Establishing earlier bedtimes for your children at every age supports a healthy mind and body. Nowadays, many children stay up late on their digital devices playing video games and chatting with friends and miss this critical window. When these patterns continue, they can create imbalances in your child's mind and body.

Aligning with Nature's Rhythms

Ayurveda has followed natural rhythms for prevention long before the Nobel Prize was awarded to scholars for discoveries on the molecular mechanisms of circadian rhythms in 2017. In fact, the science of Ayurveda has been at it for over five thousand years and recognizes the daily cycle of the doshas as it relates to both our own biological clock and to nature's rhythms. This is why it's so important to go to sleep before the pitta time of night begins at 10 p.m.—for example, so you will not have to struggle to shut down the active and sensitive state of the mind governed by the cycle of the doshas at this time. Following the same principle, the kapha time of day, between 6–10 p.m., is the preferred time to fall asleep and naturally supports the winding down of all the senses and relaxing in the evening. You will also fall asleep much easier and more quickly during this window!

Our connection with nature is vital. When you live out of sync with the rhythms and flow of nature, imbalances arise. Have you ever noticed that before the sun even rises, you start to hear the birds singing? Nature wakes up during the middle part of the vata time of the morning, 2 a.m. to 6 a.m. When the sun begins to rise, our innate nature also rises because our bodies, rhythms are connected with nature's circadian rhythms. Children tend to naturally wake up toward the end of the vata period of the morning and the beginning of the kapha period at 6 a.m. You may notice as your children get older, this timing shifts—especially in the teenage years.

If you or your children are not in alignment with nature's circadian rhythms, it may take a little time and conscious adjustment to bring the body's rhythms back into balance. Remember, the waking cycle is determined by when you go to sleep. When the sun starts to go down and the moon rises, we naturally begin to settle down, just as many animals in nature do preparing for rest. Sleep allows your body to rejuvenate itself from the day, essential not only for your precious growing children but also for you to stay healthy and balanced and in alignment with nature. The kapha time of the evening, 6 p.m. to 10 p.m., carries qualities of being heavy and slow-moving; this is the time to go with nature's flow, slow down, and settle in for the night. Since this time is governed by the energy of cohesion, it's best to eat a lighter meal to avoid feelings of heaviness and then enjoy relaxing evening routines like reading, sharing the day's events with family, and maybe even listening to some soft music. A relaxed mind and body can easily drift off to sleep before 10 p.m.

If someone's bedtime routine in your home needs adjusting, the shifts should always be gradual as extreme changes can create stress on the body system. Make any necessary time shifts in thirty- to sixty-minute increments. For example, if you have a teenager who goes to bed at 11:30 p.m., move the bedtime to 11 p.m. for a couple of weeks and then adjust it again to 10:30, and so on, until you find your child is asleep no later than 10. Once your child's sleep schedule is reset, they will naturally begin to wake up earlier.

Do your children wake up just in time to go to school and sometimes rush out of the house without even eating breakfast? This type of morning routine creates undue stress for both children and parents. Helping your children set up healthy sleep habits will get them out of bed earlier and give them time for their morning routines, prepare for school that day, have a proper breakfast, and go to school peacefully. This supports your children all day long mentally and emotionally to feel calm and balanced, be better focused on academics, and enjoy their friends and classroom activities.

Sleep and Your Child's Dosha

You will find through your everyday experiences that your children's sleep patterns are based on their doshic tendencies. In a recent article in *Psychology Today*, Ayurveda was credited as the first science to adopt "bio time" as a foundation of medicine and disease prevention and recognized for supporting sleep practices based on the doshas.[1] Following these individual guidelines can help you support and tailor healthy sleep routines based on your child's dosha.

VATA

Vata children need more sleep compared to the other doshas to avoid degeneration and depletion, though they may *want* to sleep less. Their sleep tends to be light, restless, and filled with dreams. Vata sleep imbalances often involve difficulty sleeping, teeth grinding, sleepwalking or talking, and waking up frequently—or waking during vata time from 2 to 6 a.m. These sleep disturbances can lead to feelings of anxiety and not being rested. To bring vata back into balance, Ayurveda recommends a full-body massage with warming oils like sesame oil or applying a drop of oil on the scalp and massaging the feet before bed. Offering your child a thicker blanket, or even a weighted blanket, may help with vata imbalances.

PITTA

Pitta children need consistent hours of sleep to relax and unwind because their minds are prone to intellectualization! Their sleep tends to be light, but it is easy for them to fall back to sleep if they wake up. Their mind often keeps them awake at night, which can cause difficulty sleeping, especially between 10 p.m. and 2 a.m. when sleep is essential to "digest" the day and effect cellular repair. Pitta imbalances can leave them feeling angry and sweaty. Their dreams tend to be vivid and involve problem-solving. To balance pitta, avoid stimulating activities at night, as well as caffeine and spicy food, and use coconut oil or another Ayurvedic cooling oil for body or foot massage. Don't overheat these children at night with heavy covers, especially when it's warm outside.

KAPHA

Kapha children experience the deepest sleep and so need less than other kids, though they may crave more. They generally do not dream and often want to take daytime naps, which should be avoided as they grow older. Kapha imbalances lead to daytime fatigue, daytime sleeping, and feeling groggy during the day. To balance kapha, encourage your child to get plenty of vigorous exercise and eat warm, light foods with spices. Vary their activities and massage them lightly with a warming oil before bed.

Insufficient sleep at night can cause many body mind problems in children including fatigue, constipation, low energy, attention issues, difficulty in mood regulation, falling asleep in the classroom, being unable to stay asleep, reduced social skills, and difficulty getting out of bed in the morning. It is not only a lack of sleep that can cause problems. It is important to note, especially for parents of adolescents who may want to sleep until noon that too much sleep can also cause issues such as extreme fatigue, slow digestion and metabolism, obesity, anxiety, and even memory issues.

Sleep Tips for Parents

Ayurveda considers sleep one of the pillars of life and ultimate rejuvenators of the mind and body, yet getting sound sleep is much neglected in the twenty-first century. Balanced health calls for maintaining equilibrium of building and burning, inputs and outputs, and activity and rest— in short, a dynamic harmony. Sleep is critical for the developing brain of your child and overall physical and mental well-being and facilitates that harmony through restoration, rest, and recuperation. Prioritizing your children's sleep routines supports their overall continued health and well-being and sets everyone up for a good night's sleep. Here are some sleep tips the whole family can follow!

1. Follow a routine. Do your best to ensure your children have a regular bedtime. Maintaining a set sleep schedule reminds a child's mind-body system to stay in alignment with natural circadian rhythms.
2. Encourage your children to go to sleep early and wake up early. While this may be difficult for older children and teens who tend to stay up late studying, it's a good habit to adopt that will also aid morning evacuation and leave time for breakfast.
3. Discourage teenagers trying to catch up on sleep from sleeping late on the weekends as this just makes them groggy during the day. It is important to note that too much sleep can also lead to extreme fatigue, slow digestion and metabolism, obesity, anxiety, and even memory issues. It's better to wake them up early and encourage them to take a catnap during the day if they feel depleted.

4. Set up better sleep routines for your children like taking a warm bath in the evening or giving them a loving massage.
5. Establish a relaxing bedroom environment without a TV in the room! A clean, uncluttered space with dim lighting and music or mantras playing softly in the background helps promotes relaxation. Night-lights are calming for younger children.
6. Wear comfortable, breathable fabric at night.
7. Choose bedtime stories that are uplifting and help children feel secure—perhaps a story with a moral or a short children's myth or legend! Always avoid any stimulating activities or discussions or scary stories before going to bed.
8. Avoid going to bed hungry or eating heavy meals that are difficult to digest like oily, fried, and processed foods. Drinking too much water before bedtime could mean waking up to use the bathroom; be mindful to sip water in the evening.
9. Avoid stimulating TV shows, movies, or news at least an hour before sleep.
10. Ayurveda suggests home remedies to promote sound sleep in children such as applying soothing and calming oils like Ksheerabala Thailam oil to the crown of the head and soles of the feet before bed. Wear socks to prevent slipping!
11. Offer your child an Ayurvedic sleep tonic made with whole milk and a small pinch of nutmeg (see chapter 16).
12. Breathwork and meditation enhance sleep quality. A few minutes of slow and steady Alternate Nostril Breathing or deep inhalations followed by long exhalations before bed can calm a child's mind.
13. Soothe your children's senses. This is the age of sensory and digital overload. You can help a child minimize and counterbalance these effects by not overdoing any sensory activities like overeating or staring at screens for too long. Take care of your child's sensory organs with practices such as tongue cleaning, oil massage, splashing the eyes with cool water, oil pulling (see chapter 10), and applying a couple of drops of oil in the nostrils (nasya) as recommended by your Ayurvedic professional.

14. Encourage sleeping on the left side to aid digestion.
15. It is ideal for children and adults to sleep with the head toward the south or east. Avoid sleeping with the head pointing west or north.
16. Electronic devices should be turned off or put in airplane mode. Ideally, internet modems should also be switched off when your children are sleeping. Encourage children not to stay up too late doing homework; ideally, blue light and devices should be turned off after 9 p.m.
17. Good health practices like calming yoga and exercise aid sleep. A research paper published in the *Archives of Diseases in Childhood* reported that every hour of the day kids are inactive adds three minutes to the time it takes to fall asleep; children that exercise not only fall asleep faster, they also sleep longer.[2]
18. Exercising and playing outdoors and in nature helps children unwind and relax, and improves their quality of sleep.

Some Thoughts on Co-Sleeping

Do you have a child that wants to sleep in your bed or insists you lie with them until they fall asleep? Co-sleeping is a controversial topic in America today, adopted by some and rejected by many. The Ayurvedic perspective is to co-sleep when necessary to ensure your children feel safe and can have a good night's sleep. Most children are fine sleeping on their own without any issues, but some feel very insecure and scared of the dark or of being alone in their room at night. You should always do your best to protect your child's mind from frightening experiences (as we discussed earlier when we looked at perception in chapter 7), such as scary movies or spooky Halloween events, that can easily cause nightmares when children relive these memories as they often do when alone or in a dark bedroom at nighttime.

If your child is scared and unable to sleep alone, the righteous practice for you as a parent is to provide the love and support your child needs to have a healthy night's sleep. This could mean staying with your child until they fall asleep, or maybe sleeping in your child's room for a few nights and providing some tools to help develop the confidence and courage to sleep alone. Children love sleep rituals! Saying simple prayers before bed integrating your family's faith practices, asking for blessings, and seeking protection and courage in whichever forms are meaningful to you are all very helpful to children, as is reassuring them these routines will impart safety and protection. You can find simple mantras you may like to recite with your children in chapter 11. If your child sleeps well on their own but wakes up because of a nightmare and is too scared to go back to sleep alone, give them a tight hug and invite them to enjoy sleeping with you that night. Children need love, support, and feelings of security and comfort to develop into healthy and stable adults.

9

ACTIVITY

DO YOU EVER wonder how much activity is too much activity—and if your children are overscheduled or have enough unstructured playtime or downtime to unwind mentally and physically? Between after-school activities, sports, lessons, youth clubs, and weekend commitments, it can be easy to overload—and overwhelm—your children. Sometimes, despite parents' best intentions, enriching children's lives can easily turn into depleting them, leading to burnout for the whole family.

Ayurveda considers exercise an important component of children's daily routines that provides the mental and physical benefits needed to grow up strong and healthy. Exercise enhances immunity and digestion, aids detoxification, improves mood through the release of endorphins and serotonin, lowers the risk of chronic diseases like obesity and type 2 diabetes, strengthens muscles and bones, improves sleep quality, and enhances overall confidence and feelings of self-esteem. Exercise also improves cognitive function and brain health and balances the doshas.

Balance in Motion

The key to unlocking these benefits, however, is balance—something that can be tricky for busy parents to achieve while keeping up with the hectic pace of everyday life. Ayurveda clearly conveys that exercise and activity performed beyond optimal requirements based on age, constitution, and other factors can lead to depletion and degeneration for both children and adults. We will explore the different ways Ayurveda can help you determine how much physical activity and exercise your child needs to stay healthy throughout this chapter, but just remember your intuition is key. When you notice signs of mental and physical stress, they may be overdoing things—and you may be too! Following simple Ayurvedic principles can help you customize an optimal plan of physical activity that will support your children's talents and help them develop stamina, strength, and stability.

Exercise should be performed based on your child's constitution, current imbalances, and the following considerations:

- Age: All children are in the kapha stage of life and need activities specific to their kapha age versus the elderly who are in the vata stage of life and prone to more degenerative disorders like arthritis.
- Strength: While exercise is important for building strength, it's important you follow your child's constitutional guidelines for stamina and endurance to avoid overexertion.
- Physique: Honor your child's natural body type; some children are petite, others are well-built.
- Habitat: Be mindful of the effects of the doshas where you live. Increased activity levels and water sports may be ideal near a beach, but in drier locations, you may have to be more mindful about vata aggravation and counterbalancing exercise and activity with nutrition and massage, for example.
- Season: Adapt your child's activity levels to the seasonal cycles of the doshas.

Ayurvedic Guidelines for Exercise

1. Intensity: As a rule of thumb, Ayurveda recommends exercising to half of one's capacity at a maximum, also called *balaardh*,

which helps maintain energy without undue stress or injury to any of the joints or body systems. Breaking a mild sweat is a good indication of just about enough exercise.

2. Breath: Emphasize to children they should always breathe through the nostrils and exercise with awareness to calm the nervous system. Deep breaths, abdominal breathing, and yogic breathwork support exercise routines. As endurance and tolerance increase, it will become easier and easier for your children to catch their breath during strenuous sports. When children find it difficult to breathe through their nose, this can signal physical overexertion.

3. Time of day: The ideal time to exercise is during the kapha period of the morning from 6 a.m. to 10 a.m. when the body feels stable and strong. Physical activity during these hours brings clarity and enhances strength and digestion. Also, the qualities of exercise counterbalance qualities of kapha like sluggishness and bring warmth and lightness to the body, especially important for children prone to weight gain, congestion, and sluggishness. Ideally, Ayurveda recommends avoiding exercising during pitta and vata times of day (10 a.m. to 2 p.m. and 2 p.m. to 6 p.m.). However, this is the time many children participate in after-school sports and evening games. You can help balance the effects of activity during these hours by making sure your children properly cool down, shower, unwind, and relax at home in a calm, supportive environment. Evening is a time for light exercises and stretching that promote sleep, and all strenuous exercise should be avoided.

4. Where and how often: It is generally considered best to exercise outdoors in the fresh air, exposed to nature; just be mindful of allergies and extreme temperatures. Ayurveda considers a daily, consistent exercise routine healthy for everyone, rather than irregular starts and stops. However, vata individuals can take breaks in exercise, and to a lesser extent, so can pitta types.

5. Exercise for prevention and disease management: Ayurveda uses exercise as a therapeutic tool in the recovery process of many disorders such as type 2 diabetes or depression. Anytime there is

a constitutional imbalance or injury, for example, it is important to correct the imbalance, or wait for the injury to heal before your child resumes their exercise schedule. Ayurveda's overarching principle is always to first consider and manage any medical conditions your child may have like exercise-induced asthma.

6. Times to avoid exercise: Exercise should be avoided anytime your child feels thirsty, dizzy, has indigestion, and just after eating. Your children should never exercise when they feel emotionally upset about anything. Be mindful that exercise can increase vata and should be avoided with certain vata-related illnesses; however, some conditions like constipation and anxiety can be eased by dosha-appropriate exercise. Girls should avoid strenuous exercise during their period if possible because it can throw vata-pitta out of balance. Always exercise on a light stomach or wait two to three hours after a meal.

Exercise for Your Child's Dosha

While excessive exercise is contraindicated for young children, otherwise moderate exercise is essential for your child's growth and development and can be tailored to constitution along with other daily routines.

VATA

Vata children need activities and sports that tone their mind-body systems and won't lead to overexertion and burnout. They may show variable energy, overexercising at times and underexercising at others. Often, they are drawn to creative activities like dance. A routine in terms of both time and intensity would help them. Focus on grounding, strengthening bones and muscles, preventing injury and form rather than speed.

Vata children are well-suited to slow, balancing yoga practices, walks, dancing, martial arts, lunges, squats, and sports like badminton. They should balance aerobic exercise with strength training. Rest days to unwind and recuperate are key! Oil massage and nasya (nasal application of a drop or two of sesame oil) is found to be very rejuvenating.

PITTA

Pitta children require moderate activity. They are naturally energetic and enjoy competing with others but have to be mindful not to push themselves beyond their physical limits or they can become irritable and "heat up" in an effort to achieve perfection. These children can become irate and often get upset with their teammates and may need to cool off more often than other children. Their exercise routines should be fun and relaxing! They should avoid exertion in hot, humid conditions and try to exercise in the morning or when it cools down in the evening.

Pitta types are well-suited to gardening, swimming, surfing, hiking, cycling, and sports like tennis and hockey. A relaxing yoga practice and rest days will help balance tendencies to push themselves too far and cause imbalances.

KAPHA

Kapha children have steady energy, high endurance levels, and great physical strength. They can withstand high-impact athletics and generally excel in team sports because of their warm, friendly nature that motivates and inspires teammates. Consistent, outdoor activities will improve metabolism, enhance body reflexes, and counterbalance tendencies to gain weight. Making sports fun and relieving monotony are key!

Kapha types are well-suited to gymnastics, running, cycling, rowing, and aerobic sports like soccer, basketball, tennis, and football. Signs of imbalances include lethargy, congestion, and laziness.

Seasonal Guidelines

Following seasonal variations supports your children's exercise and activity levels. Vata dominates fall and early winter, a time to slow down and fall back. Encourage your kids to take nature walks and participate in lower-impact sports like badminton and golf along with strengthening exercises. Always make sure your children bundle up against the cold qualities of vata and kapha during the late winter and early spring anytime they exercise or play outdoor sports. Spring is a time to go out biking, hiking, and play active sports. Summer marks the pitta season; enjoy water sports like swimming and recreational sports and activities that won't overheat your children. Overall, Ayurveda recommends you increase activity levels during the kapha seasons of late winter and spring, while they can be reduced a bit in other seasons.

Exercise Contraindications and Imbalances

Heavy exercise is contraindicated for children as their tissues are suppler than adults to facilitate growth and development. Intense exercise can cause overuse or repetitive stress injuries that can lead to early hardening of the tissues and have other effects on the body such as musculoskeletal disorders. Children who undergo intense training for high-intensity competitive sports may develop joint issues, exercise-induced asthma, sleep issues, fatigue, anxiety, and other vata-related disorders. This is especially true for children with vata or vata-pitta constitutions as these children are generally slender with comparatively weaker tissues. Rest and recuperation are essential for all sports-related activities and exercise programs your child participates in to prevent depletion and exercise-induced health problems.

Excessive physical activity can lead to altered taste, nausea, vomiting, dizziness, thirst, cough, dyspnea, weight loss, and heatstroke. This is particularly true in camps or boot camps where children may overexert themselves or not be carefully supervised. Adequate first aid must be provided in such places.

OVERACTIVITY

Do your children consistently come home from school telling you they're exhausted? Maybe they don't want to get into the car or complain of aches and pains—or say they just want to play? Do you wonder if you might be pushing them too hard to keep a schedule that requires a spreadsheet to track daily lessons, practices, and multiple sports teams? You can easily determine whether your child is overscheduled and engaging in too much activity by observing signs like weight loss, physical exhaustion, mental fatigue, exercise-induced asthma, dehydration, menstrual imbalances, and regular aches and pains in the body, especially in the joints.

Ayurveda offers specific guidance and simple home remedies to manage symptoms of excessive activity:

1. Rest is the most important way to recuperate.
2. Proper nutrition and hydration are the foremost remedies for recovering from excessive activity. Many children get frequent headaches from dehydration, something that can be easily avoided by drinking adequate amounts of water based on constitution and activity level. You can also try coconut water, which aids rehydration—or Ayurveda's equivalent to a sports drink: lemon water with Himalayan pink salt and sweetened to taste with unrefined cane sugar.
3. Warm milk, bone broth, and soups are some food items that can support faster recovery. Turmeric milk with a pinch of black pepper can also reduce inflammation.
4. The application of sesame oil or traditional Ayurvedic herbal oils (see chapter 16) like Murivenna oil followed by a warm shower is found to be supportive for exercise-related aches and pains.
5. Physical therapy, yoga, or Marma therapy can help recovery.

If your children are involved in high-intensity athletic exercise or part of a competitive sports team that practices three or four times a week and plays games on the weekends, it's a good idea to add a rasayana (rejuvenator) herbal supplement to their diet like Chyawanprash, *brahmi*, *yashtimadhu*, or *guduchi*. However, these herbal formulations should not be taken without the advice of a *vaidya*, or traditional Ayurvedic professional.

SIGNS OF TOO LITTLE ACTIVITY

It's important to note that too little activity is unhealthier for your child than too much activity. When your child's activity level is inadequate for their age and constitution, it can lead to problems such as obesity, lethargy, laziness, depression, metabolic and digestion-related issues, and slowing physical, mental, and emotional development. This can also lead to chronic disorders later in life.

According to Ayurveda, the triad of health is nutrition, sleep, and balanced living. For children, the third aspect, *vihara*, means lifestyle practices, including rest and activity. Building exercise into their routine along with ensuring they do not overexercise so they can stay balanced is vital. This will help your children's health today and in the years to come. Remember that as parents, modeling good lifestyle habits for your children is essential.

10

DAILY ROUTINES

ONE OF THE very first things parents learn when they have children is the importance of establishing routines—especially at bedtime! Consistent schedules throughout the day make your child feel safe and secure, build confidence, and make life at home more predictable for everyone—which lowers stress levels and allows you to find time for your own self-care. At the heart of self-care lies the Ayurvedic daily routine known as *dinacharya*.

While your own view of self-care may center around intermittent breaks of time you set aside for restful and enjoyable activities to recharge your batteries, the reality is the effects of these moments tend to be just as fleeting as the moments themselves. Ayurveda has a much wider, sustainable scope of self-care that strives to maintain and preserve health and vitality by living in alignment with the daily and seasonal rhythms of nature. Living in tune with nature allows you to align with circadian rhythms, seasonal rhythms, and the rhythm of life itself so you can lead a long, harmonious life without depletion or stagnation sustained by the flow of nature in the form of food, water, breath, and perception.

Just as day-to-day changes in your child's environment and lifestyle habits impact their mind-body system, so do shifts in nature. These influences can be either minor or major depending on your child's age, health, and constitution. The best way you can help your children stay in balance is aligning them with nature's rhythms. Once you achieve that harmony, the body will automatically begin to flow with nature. Think of it as similar to setting up your office with a proper workstation and necessary equipment to function seamlessly. In the same way, you are putting a framework in place that provides stability so your children can thrive.

Ayurvedic routines can help your child stay in harmony with nature and keep the doshas in balance. This ensures optimal growth and development, prevents health disorders, and sustains a stable and focused mind. Ayurveda views the body as a medium or tool for action and enjoyment in all areas of life. Dinacharya helps us maintain its optimum state.

The Daily Routine

Following a daily routine is like swimming with the current of a river. It helps you flow through your day in harmony with nature's rhythms and balanced mind-body functions, whereas sporadic, inconsistent lifestyle choices cause unnecessary struggles. When you teach your children the art of the daily routine, you prepare them for a life of balance, strength, and longevity.

Regardless of constitution, children need regular daily routines that align them with nature's circadian rhythms and their bodies' functional needs. Establishing routines such as going to bed early and eating at set mealtimes to maintain healthy digestion and metabolism are examples of simple ways Ayurveda can help you keep your child's constitution in balance. Understanding the daily time cycle of vata-pitta-kapha (as we saw illustrated earlier by the dosha clock in chapter 2) provides another tool you can use to support your children's lifestyle routines and activities.

Children today are tasked with handling a surplus of stimuli in their lives everywhere they go. All of this excess stimulation can lead to sensory overload and generate restlessness, hyperactivity, and anxiety—expressions of increased vata. The Ayurvedic principle of establishing daily routines creates balance and synergy with the world as it turns and helps restore doshas that have fallen out of sync with nature. Just as your body has a clock, so do the doshas! Understanding which qualities of the doshas are supportive during specific times of the day can help you learn how to support your children's daily routines and flow according to nature's wisdom and the cycles of the doshas:

2 A.M.–6 A.M. = VATA	The principle of creativity, movement, and activity; supports the meditation period of Brahma Muhurta and inner reflection; nature starts waking up; the chorus of the birds begins.
6 A.M.–10 A.M. = KAPHA	The principle of cohesion and slower movement; supports taking time for self-care during the morning routine, cleansing rituals, and eating a moderate breakfast.
10 A.M.–2 P.M. = PITTA	The principle of transformation; supports eating the largest meal of the day, productivity, and learning.
2 P.M.–6 P.M. = VATA	The principle of movement and activity; children engage in after-school sports, exercise, and studying; you may notice some restlessness as vata increases.
6 P.M.–10 P.M. = KAPHA	The principle of cohesion and slower movement; a time to settle down from the day and enjoy a lighter meal along with evening self-care rituals that prepare the body for sleep.
10 P.M.–2 A.M. = PITTA	The principle of transformation; supports the inner mind to continue subtle transformations like reconsolidation of memory while the outer mind and body are asleep.

As the sun rises and your children wake up, encourage them to drink a cup of warm water. This will kindle the digestive fire (agni) and help create a natural urge for a bowel movement, a sign of good health first thing in the morning. Encourage your children to allow this urge, but not to forcefully create the urge as this will aggravate vata and create problems in the future. It's important to note your child should follow all of their different natural urges such as urinating, sneezing, coughing, thirst, hunger, yawning, and crying, for example. Denying or holding on to these natural urges can result in vata imbalances along with specific disorders that correlate to the resisted urge. For example, holding on to the urge to have a bowel movement can cause headaches and muscle cramps.

Oral Care

Tooth brushing cleanses the mouth, strengthens the gums, kills bacteria, improves bad breath, and reduces excess kapha. Cleansing the palate first thing in the morning also helps your child enjoy all the tastes of a nourishing breakfast! Traditionally, Ayurveda uses tooth powders made from a combination of herbs such as *neem, babul, khadira,* and *karanja* for daily hygiene regimens. Nowadays, people use toothpastes, of course, many of which are formulated with ingredients that lead to sublingual absorption of chemicals. Regular use of these products causes accumulation over time and is especially unhealthy for children. The sooner you introduce your children to natural ingredients the better! Fortunately, there are many commercial toothpastes available today in natural food markets and from Ayurvedic product suppliers formulated with the recommended Ayurvedic herbs that come in refreshing flavors great for kids and adults. Teeth should be cleaned in the morning, at night, and after each meal. Exceptions to brushing are anytime your child has a throat infection, mouth ulcers, problems with the tongue, palate, or lips, or specific dental problems.

Has your child ever seen you brush your tongue or use a tongue scraper? Teaching your child to observe different textures, coatings, and cracks on their tongue can be a fun, exploratory process you can do together as part of a morning routine. Using a stainless steel or copper tongue cleaner, scrape the tongue gently after brushing the teeth. Younger children can initially brush their tongue with a soft toothbrush. This simple routine helps remove the coating from the tongue—an indication of ama—eliminates bad breath, and improves your sense of taste.

Ayurvedic texts recommend gargling or swishing with herbal teas made from simple herbs—a much better alternative to harsh commercial mouthwashes (see page 229 for an Ayurvedic mouth rinse recipe).

This practice soothes the voice, cleanses the mouth, keeps the lips moist, and can reduce tendencies to develop stomatitis—inflammation of the oral cavity. Common practices these days include completing your oral hygiene routines with herbal oils (Ayurvedic oil pulling) such as Arimedadi Thailam or a light tea made from licorice powder combined with a little raw honey—another simple recipe you can mix up with your children! Place the oil or herbal wash in the mouth after brushing and tongue scraping, then gargle or swish for a few minutes before spitting it out. Do not swallow.

Bathing

Kids get dirty! Giving your children a bath or shower once or twice a day not only cleanses the dirt and sweat from their bodies but also energizes the body, mind, and senses. Bathing improves digestion, removes lethargy, and opens the body channels for better circulation and elimination of toxins. Bathe your child in warm water unless you have a child with a pitta constitution and the weather is very hot—then milder water would be better. Hot water is always contraindicated for hair washing as Ayurveda considers direct applications of heat unhealthy for the eyes and hair. For the same reason, it's preferable to towel-dry your child's hair and scalp after a shower instead of using a hot blow-dryer. If you do use a blow-dryer, choose a cool or low setting. Take care to always make sure you thoroughly dry your child's hair as a wet scalp increases natural tendencies toward kapha disorders such as congestion and headaches.

Ideal times for bathing are in the morning after your child has a bowel movement or before a meal. If you're accustomed to bathing your children in the evening as part of a relaxing bedtime routine, do so either before dinner or an hour afterward. Bathing after a meal causes indigestion, bloating, and a delay in the downward movement of food from the stomach to the intestines and alters blood circulation necessary for the digestive process. In simpler terms, this can compromise agni and create sluggishness in your child's system. Avoid bathing your child during periods of illness.

Did you know your child's skin can eat, drink, and breathe? It may come as a surprise to some parents that paying close attention to the ingredient lists on your child's soaps, shampoos, and lotions is every bit as important as reading food labels. Every product you apply to your child's body is directly absorbed into their system. A child's skin is 30 percent thinner than adults, leaving them more vulnerable to dermal absorption of toxic chemicals lurking on the skin's surface. These exposures can lead to conditions such as cancer, nervous system damage, allergies, hormone disruption, and eczema. There are many resources available today that can help parents identify and avoid dangerous ingredients found in some children's body care products. As a general rule, avoid personal care and skincare products that contain petroleum derivatives and other chemical ingredients.

Traditionally, Ayurveda makes natural cleansing scrubs that gently remove the oils and dirt from a child's sensitive skin from the flour of lentils, chickpeas, and mung beans. This is a fun activity you can do at home with your kids that shows them how to begin creating natural skincare and beauty routines—something older children and adolescents especially love! Start by making different pastes from these simple ingredients and experimenting with varying consistencies by adding a little water or milk—especially beneficial for children who have a tendency toward dry skin. You can also add herbs such as Indian gooseberry (*amalaki*) or sandalwood powder into the pastes to enhance skin quality or even a few drops of rosewater—an Ayurvedic favorite for skincare recipes known for its softening, soothing properties and uplifting aroma.

Oil Application

Abhyanga, or oil application to the body and scalp, is considered an important daily routine for both children and adults in Ayurveda and does wonders to pacify vata, which tends to get aggravated from the day's activities. Oleation prevents dryness and degeneration, relieves tiredness, strengthens the body, improves vision, enhances nourishment, improves skin quality, and supports relaxation and sound sleep.

Not only is this a beautiful bonding experience for you and your children, but it also teaches them the importance of making time for their own self-care in the years to come. Set aside at least fifteen minutes to give your child an oil massage—the minimum amount of time it takes for the oil to be fully absorbed into the skin and strengthen and nourish the deeper tissues of the body. Afterward, your child can take a bath or shower with warm water and rinse the oil off with a natural soap or one of the homemade cleansing pastes mentioned earlier.

Chances are high you might find it difficult to work this practice into your child's routine on a daily basis—especially if your own time for self-care is limited! Your child will benefit from this loving ritual even once or twice a week, which may also create time for you to experience the benefits of abhyanga for yourself. The Sanskrit word *sneha* means both "love" and "oil." Taking the time to nurture your body with this ancient healing practice can echo the same experience and feelings of being deeply loved. Implementing this routine into your children's lives also supports them to grow up with a healthy body image and cultivate self-love and acceptance.

On the days you don't have time to give your children a whole-body massage, you can apply a few drops of oil to the soles of their feet and the crown of their head. This simple routine will cool down your child's system and promote deep relaxation and sound sleep. This traditional practice is especially beneficial for children who have disturbed sleep or trouble falling asleep. Avoid applying oil to the body or scalp if your child has a fever, cold, runny nose, or congestion and wait an additional day after symptoms resolve to resume oil applications.

AYURVEDIC HERBAL OILS

The most commonly used oil for abhyanga application in children is coconut oil, especially the virgin coconut oil made from coconut milk. Ayurveda recommends many formulated herbal oils you can use based on your child's constitution along with functional oils to support specific health needs. These include Lakshadi Thailam oil for supporting normal skeletal growth and development, joint mobility, and optimal function of the nervous system. Nalpamaradi Keram oil is popular for its skincare properties, a classic formulation known to maintain radiant, soft, and illuminated skin. This particular oil is also used to treat a wide range of skin infections such as pruritus, scabies, and eczema and for skin irregularities like uneven skin tone and blemishes. You will find common therapeutic and massage oils you can select according to your child's dosha in the table at the end of chapter 16. Deciding which herbal-infused oils are best for your child can easily be assessed with your vaidya or Ayurvedic practitioner.

Hair and Scalp Care

The key principles to keeping your child's scalp and hair healthy are to maintain moisture or slight oiliness on the scalp as well as avoiding hot showers and hair dryers. Regular oil application to the scalp not only keeps hair lustrous and healthy but can improve sleep quality, support and maintain good vision, improve focus, and calm the mind. It can also strengthen the bones of the skull, prevent headaches, and sharpen the senses.

One of the most rejuvenating hair and scalp care oils is Kesini oil, formulated from a unique base of freshly pressed castor and coconut oils along with *bacopa* (brahmi), hibiscus, and Indian gooseberry (*amalaki*). This tonic revitalizes, moisturizes, and nourishes the scalp and hair roots and maintains the hair's natural color and texture. Kesini oil also helps regulate blood circulation to hair follicles and promotes luster and shine. The usual method is to apply oil to the scalp using gentle massage and keep it on for at least fifteen to twenty minutes before washing it out. Other specific oils for scalp application suggested in Ayurveda are in chapter 16.

Nose and Ear Care

Adopting the practice of oil application, or nasya, in your child's nose and ear care routines helps to strengthen the mind and body. Children above the age of seven can apply a drop of Anu Thailam oil in each nostril once a day using a nasal dropper, a practice known to help stabilize the mind and emotions. Ayurveda considers nasya a doorway to the brain, the location of all the centers of the sense organs and organs of action. As part of a daily routine, nasya enhances sensory acuity, improves immune resistance, sharpens the sense organs, and prevents diseases above the neck such as sinus problems, migraines, headaches, and neck stiffness. It strengthens the joints in the scalp and face and improves the texture of the skin and clarity of the voice.

To perform nasya at home, have your child lie down with their head tilted back slightly as you administer one drop of warm oil into each nostril, then ask them to lightly sniff. Should any oil come into the throat or mouth, have them spit it out and try not to swallow it. Nasya should not be performed within an hour of eating, and there should be at least thirty minutes between nasya practice and bathing.

According to Ayurveda, the ear is a vata-predominant sense organ, and regular oil application can help pacify vata and associated disturbances of the ear. Ayurvedic ear care can be especially helpful to improve hearing and prevent ringing in the ears. This practice also loosens earwax, strengthens the ear bones and eardrums, and prevents neck stiffness. Simply instill a few drops of warm sesame oil or Anu Thailam in both of your child's ears. This can be done at the same time as nasya since your child will already be lying down. For earaches, garlic or clove oil is traditionally used. Try to avoid exposing your children to loud music and noises. You can also keep cold air from rushing into your child's ears by placing small cotton balls inside the ears during cold weather—a popular tip among parents!

Ayurveda is in no way a prescriptive science. It is a system of principles and guidelines to help support a long, healthy life that you can choose to integrate in whichever ways work best. There is no rule that says you must adopt every one of these lifestyle practices or daily routines. In fact, that would cause undue feelings of stress—exactly what Ayurveda strives to counterbalance! How much should you do? You should do as much or as little as is practically possible given your life circumstances, and focus on the practices you feel will most benefit your children.

The key philosophy in Ayurveda is that making even small changes to your lifestyle can create significant positive shifts. Your intention to make positive changes in your child's life—no matter how many or few—becomes the reflection of your true love and care as a parent. Simplicity and consistency are two watchwords for positive health. Taking simple, small steps consistently is better than striving for monumental changes occasionally!

11

YOGA, MEDITATION, AND MANTRAS FOR KIDS

MOST CHILDREN ARE natural-born yogis. You see it yourself every day—your kids monkeying around everywhere, mimicking animals, bridges, trees and twisting themselves up into pretzels! Even from the time they're infants, you can notice their thumb and index finger touching lightly in Chin Mudra or thumb cozily tucked in the other fingers in Chinmaya Mudra, both of which naturally help development of the brain. As your children grow, their spontaneous play and frolicking is a lot like yogic postures or asanas in a fun, unstructured, manner!

However, much like you, the demands of modern life gradually lead them to unnatural body positions hunching over a computer with tightened shoulders or walking bent over and sideways carrying an overloaded backpack to school. Add in decreased physical activity and you can see how easy it is for them to forget their innate nature.

When your children adopt yoga, breathwork, meditation, and mantras into their lives, they grow up healthier and happier and continue these practices into adulthood.

Now that yoga has become popular everywhere, many parents today are eager to explore these different postures and techniques at home with their families. Maybe you even have a yoga practice of your own you'd like to share with your kids—or even better, start one together with them! Many children today have been introduced to yoga and simple meditation exercises in school and, thanks to initiatives like the Mindful Schools Curriculum that empower educators to cultivate awareness and resilience with compassionate action in education, students across the United States are being nurtured and supported socially, emotionally, and academically in "mindful schools" and learning environments. A growing body of research demonstrates the integration of mindfulness programs led by qualified teachers helps children thrive not only in the classroom with improved attention and focus, emotional regulation, and social skills, but also with reducing feelings of stress at home and enhanced well-being.[1]

Yoga and Ayurveda

Yoga and Ayurveda are sister sciences that emanate from the Vedas and share the same goal of seeking balance between mind, body, and spirit to prevent disease and live life to its fullest potential. While many people today use yoga as a popular way to enhance their fitness routines, its therapeutic context is essentially Ayurvedic in nature, and traditionally it was meant as a spiritual practice, or *sadhana*, for managing the mind. In fact, Ayurveda is the earliest known medical science to recommend exercise, or *vyayama*, for preventive health and disease management. Ayurveda recommends yoga asanas to enhance physical and mental health and well-being, raise consciousness, and restore balance to the doshas.

In Ayurvedic terms, these practices help to calm, energize, and integrate body, mind, and spirit. You can adopt yoga as part of an Ayurvedic protocol to help eliminate accumulated or imbalanced doshas from deeper tissues and aid removal of excess vata and ama—toxins that may have accumulated in bones and joints. Yoga postures and sequences balance all of the doshas, promote longevity, aid rejuvenation, and enhance awareness. They also balance the energy centers in your subtle body, known as *chakras*.

Despite popular belief, yoga is not merely the practice of body postures and sequential movements (asanas) or stretches, but encompasses a personal and societal ethic, breathwork, and meditation. Many people are surprised to learn that yoga has eight limbs, each its own unique principle to cultivate a life expressing the highest human potential at all levels—physical, mental, emotional, social, and spiritual. The purpose of cultivating this alignment and oneness within yourself and with all of creation is to unleash your inner potential as a human being. While some of these practices need to be introduced gradually to children, like advanced asanas or breathwork, it is very important to seed the right principles and practices, no matter what their age—and it's never too early or late to start! A child's yoga practice can have innumerable benefits and help children feel calm, balanced, and aligned with their own mind-body consciousness as well as the world around them. Below are the eight limbs of yoga you may want to research independently as your knowledge of Ayurveda deepens:

- *Yama* (practices toward the environment and community like nonviolence)
- *Niyama* (practices for ourselves like cleanliness and contentment)
- *Asana* (postures and sequential movements)
- *Pranayama* (breathwork)
- *Pratyahara* (withdrawal of senses)
- *Dharana* (concentration)
- *Dhyana* (meditation)
- *Samadhi* (complete integration and living in a meditative or enlightened state)

In the same way you can adapt your children's lifestyle routines to their prakriti or *vikriti* (current state of imbalance), you can also tailor yoga practices to support and balance the doshas. Ayurveda's adaption of yoga and other tools is based on balancing subtle energies in the body and integrating knowledge of yoga postures and different actions of the breath into daily routines for mental and physical healing and well-being. For chronic health conditions, yoga is adapted to balance the doshas and reduce the risk of any further complications or injury. Just as you can stabilize the body through a physical practice, you can also stabilize the mind. When you strive to balance the doshas with the complementary practices of yoga and Ayurveda, you can also balance the *trigunas*, or the qualities of mind we discussed in chapter 7. Practicing yoga can reduce tamas or lethargy, balance rajas or feelings of restlessness and aggression, and enhance sattva, a clear, calm, light, productive, and happy state of mind. Yoga, breathwork, and meditation work together to help restore children to their prakriti, or state of individual homeostasis and health. The knowledge of your child's constitution and tendencies you've learned from previous chapters along with an awareness of the trigunas can help you specifically tailor your child's yoga practice to the doshas, as we will discuss later in this chapter.

BENEFITS OF YOGA

Yoga, breathwork, meditation, and mantra are all tools you can use to help your children feel deeply grounded and aligned with the universe. This promotes peace, health, and harmony both on and off the yoga mat! Sharing these lifestyle therapies as a family is also a wonderful way to bond with your children and show them how special they are to you. Maybe you have more than one child. For parents looking for ways to create quality time to spend individually with their children, simple yoga sequences are the perfect way to be present and playful. Fifteen minutes of one-on-one time can be especially meaningful for a child who has siblings. Following is a list of the ways your children can benefit from yoga, breathwork, and meditation:

- Stress management: Children move from the flight and freeze mode (sympathetic nervous system) to the rest and digest mode (parasympathetic nervous system)
- Increased focus
- Improved mental health; reduction of anxiety, depression, and eating disorders
- Enhanced physical health, digestion, and metabolism
- Improved academic performance at school
- Improved memory and cognition

- Increased creativity and lateral thinking
- Improved sleep
- Boosted self-awareness and self-esteem
- Promotion of attitudes of compassion and cooperation rather than competitiveness
- Breaking free from digital media and overscheduling, which soothes the eyes, sensory organs, and mind
- Managing specific conditions such as indigestion, headaches, autism, and ADHD
- Reduced behavioral issues
- Improved immunity and vitality
- Better physical and mental flexibility and strength
- Healthy habits to carry into adulthood that aid quality of life and longevity
- Resilience to cope with stressors in a healthy and productive way

Yoga Sequences for Children

Yoga sequences are combinations of primary postures that include Sun Salutations, standing poses, seated poses, and balancing postures. Each of these asanas has physical and mental effects. For example, Vajrasana (the Diamond Pose or Thunderbolt) is a very common asana practice known to improve the stability and tone of knee joints, legs, and thighs and used as a tool to manage lower back issues. It is also an asana that supports meditation practices as it provides the perfect geometry for optimum body stability and facilitates relaxation, concentration, and complete peace of mind. Generally, balancing poses require attention, increase lung function, and generate heat, while standing postures are weight-bearing and bring strength and stability. Seated poses are the most stable yoga poses and enhance groundedness and concentration. Sun Salutations are practiced as a flow of various asanas that will bring optimal flexibility, strength, and physical alignment to the body.

Knowing your child's constitution along with the basic understanding of the doshas you now have can help you adapt these complementary practices to your child's unique nature and keep pace with their changing day-to-day needs. Understanding the fundamental anatomy of the doshas adds another helpful layer of information when preparing to introduce yoga sequences to your children. According to Ayurveda, the seat of kapha is the chest and upper clavicle region, the seat of pitta the abdomen, and the seat of vata the lower abdominal region below the navel, particularly the colon.

Keeping the fundamental qualities of the doshas in mind can help you choose the best yoga postures and sequences to keep your children in balance and create your own along the way! As you know, kapha and vata require warmth to maintain balance while pitta requires cooling. Here are some general principles to refer to when selecting asanas for your child. Please be aware the same postures can become heating or cooling depending on the effort, speed, and duration of the practice.

Generally, supine poses on the back are relaxing while prone positions on the belly are more dynamic and heating. Seated poses like forward bends or rotating postures are considered balancing for vata by releasing blocked energy, and inverted postures can be both heating and cooling but are great for kapha. Forward bends release tension from the mid-abdomen region where pitta accumulates, and twists can be heating but also aid digestion and release accumulated pitta. Backbends generally kindle agni but must be done carefully by vata types to avoid injuries. Restorative poses generate heat and can be supported by a range of different props. You'll find simple yoga sequences for younger children and teens on the following pages, but first here are some yoga tips for parents:

A PLAYFUL PRACTICE: Kids love fun and games! Get things moving with yoga freeze dance and ask children to strike their favorite yoga pose (or make one up) every time the music stops. Be prepared for lots of giggling! Another yoga game is to challenge children to run across the room to music and pause when you call out different postures like Tree Pose, for example. The children who can hold the poses continue with the game and whoever reaches the end of the room first gets to decide the next posture kids have to hold or pick the next game.

BE FLEXIBLE: Kids are not as disciplined as adults, so allow for fidgeting, giggling, goofing around, nonparticipation, breaks, and imperfection.

Relate to them with humor while setting appropriate limits, especially to avoid injuries.

TRY CREATIVE TECHNIQUES: Animal yoga and partner yoga are two great options. Kids love Cat and Cow Pose and will often meow or moo along making funny sounds and imitating different kinds of animals. They love variations too; your Butterflies can sway in the wind just as your Trees can! Children will enjoy partnering up with friends and the challenge of creative directions.

AN ACTIVE PRACTICE: As kids get older and into their teens, it helps to make the practice very active so it can dissipate energy and reduce rajas.

AVOID POWER STRUGGLES AND LEAD BY EXAMPLE! Parenting is often about picking your battles, and a yoga practice that is meant to relax everyone shouldn't be one of them. Model positive resolve by doing your own yoga regularly, even if it's only a short practice . . . especially if all you have time for is a very, very short practice! When you take care of yourself, you are better able to take care of your kids.

A SAMPLE YOGA SEQUENCE FOR YOUNGER CHILDREN

- Warm-up with jumping jacks or jogging in place. If they are in a group setting, one child can be the leader and do a fun warm-up others can follow.
- Standing balancing poses like Tree, Warrior, and Chair to transition to sitting and seated poses
- Alternatively, if they are little older, Sun Salutations
- Cat and Cow Pose
- Transition to Downward Dog, Cobra, and then Child's Pose
- Sit up for Butterfly, Mill Churning, Camel
- On their back, Boat and Wind Releasing Pose (you may hear giggling!)
- On their stomach, Locust, Cobra, Flying Super Person, and Bow Pose

- Lie on their backs for Shavasana, or final relaxation—a time you can build in some affirmations and guided imagery

- Seated rotations
- Cat and Cow
- Downward Dog
- Transition to Standing Forward Bend
- Warrior 1, 2, and 3
- Triangle
- Twisting
- Sun Salutations for a few rounds
- Chair Pose
- Similar sequence as younger children on back (add cycling) and belly
- Shavasana or final relaxation can be longer

YOGA FOR YOUR CHILD'S DOSHA

Now that you have viewed your child and their tendencies through an Ayurvedic lens, you are probably eager to learn more about the ways you can use yoga to support your child's unique constitution. Here, we'll explore principles that will help you customize your child's yoga practice to keep the doshas aligned and counterbalance disease tendencies.

o o o

A pitta child may be prone to anger or jealousy as an imbalance and may overdo exercise. A vata child may be restless and lacking in focus. A kapha child may have a tendency to be lazy.

o o o

Vata needs regular, grounding, slow, and warming yoga, which is restorative, gentle, and at less than their capacity. Vata children are drawn to variety and overdoing things, but most of all need routine and consistency. Though these children naturally crave a fast pace, it helps if they slow down and hold poses for a bit longer than they may be inclined. Emphasize warming, circulating, and downward movement of energy with standing poses held for about three breaths. A slow even breathing rhythm keeps vata balanced and ensures good flow of prana. Poses that are especially beneficial for them are floor sequences, seated and standing forward bends, gentle backbends, twisting (which aids their variable digestion), Tree Pose, Mountain Pose, and a long, slow relaxation to end the practice.

Pitta may be drawn to intense and heating yoga, which is competitive with their tendency toward perfectionism (especially for teenagers), which they need to counterbalance. These children need slow, relaxing, nurturing, gentle movements with an emphasis on noncompetitive yoga. Forward bends are cooling and spinal twists help disperse built-up heat and tension from the stomach and small intestines. (Take care during backbends and spinal compression not to overdo things.) Seated and lying twists soothe pitta, and overall twisting performed with lunging or kneeling is very soothing. Slow Sun Salutations are great—just make sure your children are practicing in a cool environment or at a cool time of day, preferably before sunrise or in the evening.

Kapha needs to rev up their routine and have an energetic practice they can easily switch around to break up monotony! Kapha children may resist the practice but are actually very strong constitutionally, and this will help activate their mind-body system and ensure they don't slip into laziness. A warmer, faster-paced class that stimulates respiration, increases circulation, and induces sweating is especially good for them. Kapha constitutions should minimize floor asanas that can lead to feelings of lethargy and wanting to take a short nap! Fast-paced Sun Salutations and standing and supported or modified inverted poses are very beneficial.

CONTRAINDICATIONS AND GUIDELINES

Yoga is a health practice and, often, a therapeutic tool. It is important to ensure your children learn yoga in a class or studio from a trained practitioner at least initially in your presence to avoid injuries.

Because children are naturally so much more flexible than adults, it's important to be especially mindful they don't overextend their joints or push themselves if they feel any type of pain. Anytime children are practicing yoga in a group, keep enough space between them to ensure they don't bump into each other and cause injuries, and keep the group to a manageable size. Always remember to counter poses and avoid overstretching or overextending muscles, ligaments, and tendons. Easier poses are a good place to begin before moving on to more challenging ones as children have to build strength and stability before beginning advanced yoga practices. The duration of the practice should not be so long that younger kids get fidgety and unfocused, which can increase their propensity to get injured. A children's yoga teacher will be aware of all of these concerns.

CHILDREN 3–10 YEARS OLD

- Children under ten should wait up to ten seconds and take a couple of breaths before transitioning into the next pose. The total time for a child's yoga session should not be more than twenty minutes.
- Children are advised not to perform asanas for long durations of time or any practices at all that require holding the breath.
- Yoga for children involves gentle stretches and movements, often mimicking animals and incorporating games.
- Imaginative stories about yoga practices are the best methods of teaching yoga to kids.
- Always demonstrate the posture, rather than explaining it. Use the same method when trying to correct poses during practical sessions.
- Avoid extreme forward- and backward-bending asanas.
- Avoid headstands and handstands.
- Avoid overstretching or pushing too hard.
- Yogic practice should be done on an empty or light stomach.
- Children should practice yoga under the supervision of an expert/trained yoga teacher with proper guidance and never alone.
- If a child complains of any discomfort during or after practice,

they should be given full attention and medical help, if needed.

- Never compare children with each other.
- Teach yoga with affection and deal with all types of reactions tenderly.
- Basic principles of yoga like *yama* and *niyama* should be emphasized while teaching yoga postures to get better results.

ADOLESCENTS UP TO 18 YEARS OLD

- There should be no feelings of competition while practicing yoga.
- Girls should avoid yoga practices during menstruation or focus on a relaxing practice.
- Yoga sequences should gradually progress from basic to more advanced poses to build strength, endurance, and flexibility over time and avoid stress and strain to the muscles and joints. Poses should be followed by pranayama, relaxation, and meditation.
- Asanas should not be practiced in haste or by applying any sort of undue force under any circumstances.
- Attain final positions step-by-step and maintain with eyes closed for an inward awareness within the whole body.
- Maintenance of the final asana is always beneficial as per one's capacity.
- Yogic practice should be done on an empty or light stomach.
- Duration of time and awareness spent in postures can gradually increase as children transition from childhood to adulthood.
- Adolescents often have a negative body image due to bodily or hormonal changes. Teach with all such considerations in mind, encouraging them as needed.
- Physical movements from one posture to another provide strength, endurance, and flexibility to joints and muscles of growing adolescents.
- Explain what they are doing by telling teens about each practice and how the practice will be beneficial for them. Create a conducive atmosphere for them so that they can share their experiences without any hesitation.[2]

The U.S. National Institutes of Health provide additional guidelines taking into account developmental considerations in a yoga class for children and adolescents.

Age	Duration
Preschool age (3–6 years)	Total duration: 15–20 minutes Focused awareness: 2–3 minutes Poses: 10 minutes Breathing or singing: 2–3 minutes Guided visualization: 2–3 minutes
School age (7–12 years)	Total duration: 30–45 minutes Focused awareness: 3–5 minutes Poses: 15–25 minutes (can be incorporated into a story or game) Breathing or singing: 3–5 minutes Guided visualization/relaxation: 5 minutes
Adolescent (13–18 years)	Total duration: 45–90 minutes Focused awareness: 5–10 minutes Poses: 30–50 minutes Breathing: 5–10 minutes Guided relaxation: 5–10 minutes

Age	Special Considerations
Preschool and school age	Use English nature names for poses. Use short and simple instructions. Demonstrate poses. Hold poses for a maximum of 3 breaths. Maintain an attitude of playful calm. Create a safe environment.
Adolescent	Be sensitive to body image. Use touching adjustments with care; give opportunity to opt out of being touched. Be aware of clothing issues (tight jeans, bare feet, revealing shirts or shorts). Encourage a nonjudgmental and noncompetitive practice.

Meditation

Meditation is one of the unique tools used in Ayurveda to facilitate harmony and healing in the mind, body, and consciousness. The word *meditation* is used nowadays to describe many different techniques including concentration, contemplation, guided meditation, breathing exercises, mantra, and meditative movement practices like yoga or even walking meditation. While all these methods operate on diverse mind-body systems such as the senses, mind, emotions, and intellect, the true objective of meditation is to connect oneself with the soul or deep inner self. All practices that achieve this goal serve its true purpose.

Research on structured meditation programs for children and adolescents suggests a myriad of benefits relating to mental and physical health, coping skills, self-regulation, and decreased negative classroom behavior and hyperactivity. Studies of school-based mindfulness instruction have demonstrated improved psychological functioning, behavior, and focus and reduction of ADHD symptoms along with reduced levels of stress, anxiety, and depression, all from simple breathing awareness just a few minutes a day.[3]

The physical benefits of meditation include calming the nervous system, improving immunity, aiding digestion, and relieving headaches and pain. All meditation practices enhance sattva and are deeply restful for the mind, body, and spirit. Even a few minutes a day spent meditating with your children lead, to better physical, mental, and emotional health. While there are various types of meditation techniques, here are some that are easy to practice with children:

- Guided meditation or imagery is a wonderful technique in complementary therapy that allows children and adolescents to follow along with instructions on an app or video or with a practitioner. Used as a therapeutic intervention, it can help psychological functioning, reduce stress, and aid pain management. Be cautious if there is a history of PTSD and consult a mental health practitioner.
- Guided relaxation and Yoga Nidra: This is similar to the final resting pose done in yoga when you slowly bring attention to different

parts of the body from head to toe and progressively focus the breath to induce a relaxation response. When lying down, this can be done as a guided practice of progressive and deep relaxation.

- Mindfulness is a well-known technique generally practiced sitting with closed eyes and bringing one's attention to the breath. When the attention drifts away, the instruction is to bring it back without judgment. This does not require any training or years of practice. However, we have to ensure that the duration is age appropriate.

- Prayer and mantra meditation is a simple way for kids to meditate in the morning or at bedtime and can include focusing on a simple prayer or repeating a mantra like Om. A 2012 study showed that mantra meditation can improve brain health and enhance cognitive function as well as visuospatial and verbal memory. Another research project in 2017 demonstrated that chanting certain mantras may stimulate these effects by helping to synchronize the left and right sides of the brain and promote relaxing alpha brain waves.[4]

MEDITATION TIPS FOR KIDS AND TEENS

- Meditation is about relaxation. Kids are so programmed to succeed that it is a good idea to help them relax and meditate effortlessly with praise.
- Having thoughts during meditation is natural. Encourage children of all ages not to judge their thoughts, but merely observe them.
- Yoga, exercise, and breathwork all help in reducing the state of rajas or restlessness and help kids relax.
- Create an atmosphere for children that is quiet and appealing without distractions.
- Length of time and frequency of meditation should vary. Pediatricians normally recommend that preschool children meditate a few minutes per day, grade school children 3–10 minutes once or twice daily, and teens and adults 5–45 minutes per day based on their preference.

- Vata tends to be restless and may be drawn to meditation that has movement involved: guided imagery, mantra meditation, and breathing meditation.

- Pitta also does well with guided imagery; cooling mudras, water imagery, mindfulness, and loving-kindness meditations to let go of anger and resentment.

- Kapha benefits from active breathing followed by meditation to support clarity of thought and relieve dullness.

Mantras

Mantra practices center the mind utilizing a sound, phrase, or word chanted either silently in the mind or out loud. Mantra meditation is an essential practice in various types of yoga and assists to deepen inner consciousness. Traditionally, children are taught prayers growing up based on their faith. In the same way, Sanskrit chants have been taught to children in Vedic cultures right from an early age.

Mantras can be defined as the yoga of sound or thought of as asanas for the mind that use the vibrations of sound therapy to heal and balance physiology and emotions. Mantra chanting can induce a calm, meditative effect, help children feel grounded, and improve vagal tone. Mantra meditation is extremely useful for harnessing active minds and bodies—calming pitta, clearing kapha lethargy, and alleviating vata imbalances.

Mantras and chants for children can be positive affirmations, prayers, or intentions that can be recited aloud or in their minds and can be in any language (Sanskrit, Latin, Gurmukhi, Arabic, Pali, or Hebrew, to name a few). The primordial sound OM, a universal mantra, is akin to mantras and prayers from other traditions, such as *Amen, Ameen*, and *Shalom*. Following are some Sanskrit mantras children can practice daily. In cases where children may be too young to chant more complex mantras, the usual practice in traditional Ayurvedic households is for parents to play the mantras softly in the background so children can benefit from the sound vibrations.

Children might also enjoy chanting mantras in the morning or evening at bedtime. Ayurveda suggests chanting in multiples of three, a number that connects us to the past, present, and future; the three layers of existence of the physical, subtle, and causal; the three cosmic qualities of sattva, rajas, and tamas; and the three doshas. The traditional method for counting mantras in Ayurveda is the *mala*—a string of prayer beads. Children may wish to use a sandalwood, lotus seed, or pearl mala if this appeals to them and chant either silently or aloud.

OM MANI PADME HUM

OM MANI PADME HUM is the six-syllabled Sanskrit mantra specifically associated with the Bodhisattva of Compassion. The first word, *Om,* is a sacred syllable. *Mani* means bead or jewel. *Padme* is the lotus flower, and *Hum* symbolizes the spirit of enlightenment. Thus, *Om Mani Padme Hum* means that based on the practice of a path, which is an inseparable union of method and wisdom, a person can transform their mind, body, and speech into the pure, pleasant, and elevated state of being.

GAYATRI MANTRA

The Gayatri mantra is a universal prayer from the Vedas and refers to the innate and inspiring higher self—"that from which all is born." First the Gayatri, "the spirit behind the sun," is praised, then meditated upon and channeled to purify and elevate the intellect and ability to discern truth and untruth. The Gayatri mantra is recognized as the essence and true knowledge of the Vedas and cultivates and hones the ability to acquire knowledge:

OM BHUR BHUVAH SVAH
TAT SAVITUR VARENYAM
BHARGO DEVASYA DHIMAHI
DHIYO YO NAH PRACHODAYAT

We meditate on the glory of the creator who has created the three-dimensional universe with the past, present, and future, who is the embodiment of true knowledge and intellect, who is the remover of all darkness and ignorance and promotes illumination within.

Regularly chanting this mantra can help establish and calm the mind, and in turn lead to happiness and success in life. The Gayatri is a declaration of gratitude, to both the nurturing sun and the spirit.

SHANTI MANTRAS

Shanti literally translates to "peace," and the Shanti mantras are intended to establish peace and calm at all levels. There are many such peace chants from the ancient Indian teachings, the most popular being from the Brihadaranyaka Upanishad, an ancient Hindu spiritual text:

OM ASATO MA SAT GAMAYA
TAMASO MA JYOTIR GAMAYA
MRUTYORMA AMRUTAM GAMAYA
OM SHANTI SHANTI

The exact meaning of this mantra is "Lead me from the untruth to the truth, lead me from the darkness to light, lead me from mortality to immortality, and let peace prevail everywhere."

Young children can also recite the shorter mantra: OM SHANTI SHANTI. Another simple mantra for children is AHAM PREMA, a chant that invokes self-love, literally translating to "I am divine love."

MAHAMRITYUNJAYA MANTRA

The Mahamrityunjaya Mantra is a verse from the Rig Veda—the earliest of the Vedas—imparting longevity, protecting one from tragedies, and preventing premature death. This powerful mantra is known to remove fears and heal the entire mind-body system.

OM TRYAMBAKAM YAJAMAHE SUGANDHIM PUSHTIVARDHANAM
URVARUKAMIVA BANDHANAAN MRUTYORMUKSHEEYA
MAAMRUTAAT

This mantra translates as "I worship the three-eyed form of Shiva, who is fragrant and who nourishes all like the fruit falls off from the bondage of the stem, may we be liberated from death, from mortality."

Remember, you can play these mantras softly for your children if they seem difficult to recite.

Mantras work at different levels within our consciousness based on both the meaning of the mantra and the subtle sound vibrations created by the mantra.

Dr. J has seen firsthand the many ways mantras can help transform individuals and support healing. He still remembers a twelve-year-old boy from Tamilnadu in India who came for a consultation when he was working as the chief medical officer of Ayurvedagram in Bangalore. His parents brought him for an Ayurvedic consultation to help with bed-wetting, nightmares, and anxiety after they had tried other treatment modalities including modern psychiatry. After a comprehensive consultation along with suggestions of herbs and dietary and lifestyle routines, he also recommended the mantra chant "OM HANUMATE NAMAHA" and asked the boy to chant this mantra eleven times at night before he went to sleep. He also told him the story of Hanuman, the son of wind, and how powerful chanting this mantra is to remove all fears and negative occurrences. The entire family was very grateful to report their son never had any issues after starting the herbs and chanting the mantra every night. Growing up, Dr. J saw his own grandmother suggesting this mantra throughout his childhood to many parents for removing fears and anxiety in their children.

The classic texts of Indian origin record the influence of mantras on both plants and animals, and Ayurveda also recognizes the importance of this realm of medicine. The author of a particular study recording various experiments on plants found that from the stage of seedling to maturity, they were affected by certain types of sound waves, especially mantras. The study revealed that plants have shown a positive response to the particular sound frequency of chanting mantra relative to growth and efficacy curing diseases.[5]

Whether recited, whispered, or meditated upon, the rhythmic vibrations and tones of all kinds of chants can be healing and have the power to help us feel healthier, energized, and positive-minded.

Mantra therapy is one of Ayurveda's main tools for calming the mind. Two types of mantras are employed: Bija (or seed) mantras and Shakti mantras. Seed mantras are pure, simple sounds that resonate in the body at a particular frequency and activate individual chakras or energy centers of the body. Each of the Bija mantras correlates to the seven chakras, and each of the chakras has an associated dosha. Chanting particular seed sounds is another way you can support the doshas. For instance, chanting the Bija mantra Lam activates the Muladhara or root chakra and related vata dosha. As mentioned earlier, Shakti mantras are related to kindness and can enhance prana, and Prana mantras like So Hum ("I am that") increase sattva.

A child with healthy habits will grow up to be a healthier adult. Conversely, when kids suffer from physical and mental health issues, these can often linger into adulthood and cause many chronic disorders. Early experiences create biological memories while toxic stress undermines the body's stress response, brain development, cardiovascular system, immune system, and metabolic controls. What better legacy can you provide your children than the tools and techniques of yoga, breathwork, meditation, and mantras to bring them inner peace, grounding, good health, and a calm state of mind? These practices can lead them to a path of resilience they can rely on as they grow older!

PART FOUR

Understanding and Managing Common Childhood Ailments and Disorders

12

HEALTH AND DISEASE

WHEN YOUR CHILDREN get sick, do you immediately wonder who they were exposed to that had a cold or virus or where they went that was filled with germs? If you believe your children's illnesses come from picking up new pathogens and bacteria that compromise their immune system, you are looking at the situation through the modern medical lens that views health and disease as two different entities. From the Ayurvedic perspective, all disease is the outcome of deviations from within the normal structure or function—or sometimes both the structure and the function—of our own mind-body systems.

According to Ayurveda, a state of balance among the mind-body system represents health, whereas imbalance or disharmony represents disease. They are two sides of the same coin. Let's look at some examples that will lay the groundwork to help you understand how disease develops from the Ayurvedic perspective.

Two Sides of the Same Coin

The root cause of disorders and disease is always an imbalance within your own system. For example, normal and balanced blood sugar levels are an indication of health as they support normal energy requirements and vitality, whereas low blood sugar (hypoglycemia) or high blood sugar (hyperglycemia) are considered disease. Both conditions are deviations from your own normal, balanced state. In the same way, a person's ability to sustain a normal body weight is healthy, but being overweight or obese is considered disease, just as being underweight. Cholesterol is the fundamental construction unit of our cells similar to brick and cement as building materials. When cholesterol increases above certain limits, doctors will insist you take statins because your cholesterol is now in a pathological state. The same can be said of all diseases whether obesity, high cholesterol, ADHD, fevers, constipation, diarrhea, and asthma—all are aberrations from the balance within your own body.

When your children fall ill and get a fever, their rising temperature is generated by their own bodies as a response to crisis. While you may look to the transmittal of a viral or bacterial infection as the culprit, the reality is your children are constantly exposed to bacteria, viruses, fungi, and many other pathogens in their environment all the time. It is their immune resistance that prevents them from getting infections. When your child's immune system is compromised due to physical, mental, nutritional, or environmental reasons, the same pathogens they have already been exposed to attack different body systems and cause infection. Pathogens won't be able to cause infection unless your child's immune resistance is weak.

Have you ever experienced times during the school year when you found out that your child's classmates were sick and then waited for your child to come home with a fever or cold, but they never did? In cases like this, you can see that exposures to bacteria on their own do not mean your child will necessarily become ill. The strength of your child's immune system is the gatekeeper holding harmful pathogens at bay. These are a couple of different ways you can understand that health and disease are two sides of the same coin—the balanced side being a state of health, and the imbalanced side, a state of disease.

Ayurvedic Principle of Nidana

If all disease is the expression of imbalances within your child's own structures and physical and mental body functions, what causes these deviations? To understand the ways disease manifests, you need to know the different types of diseases your child can have, and from there, you can identify the root or origin of the disease—known as *nidana*. According to Ayurveda, there are seven distinct classifications of disease according to different criteria.

HEREDITARY DISEASES: The seed potential of disease existed at the time of inception and was inherited from either the maternal or paternal side. The imbalance was carried forward through one of the parent's genes. Examples of inherited disorders include muscular dystrophy, sickle cell anemia, diabetes, and cystic fibrosis.

CONGENITAL DISEASES: Disease developed during the fetal period in the mother's womb due to etiological factors including dietary, lifestyle, or psychological imbalance, or habits like smoking during the period of pregnancy. Disease tendencies generated from the intrauterine environment include hypertension, diabetes, metabolic disorders, and respiratory and mental disorders.

DISORDERS DEVELOPED DURING BIRTH AND DELIVERY: Examples include Erb's palsy and umbilical cord trauma, which can affect oxygen flow and lead to brain damage.

ACQUIRED DISEASES: These diseases are the outcome of exposures in the world after birth and are generated from dietary, lifestyle, and environmental factors that cause development of various disorders. Examples include unwholesome practices such as overeating, vaping, or smoking.

DISEASES DUE TO TIME CYCLES: Disease develops during or because of influences of various time cycles such as diurnal cycles, lunar cycles, seasonal cycles, and life cycles. Children, for example, are prone to seasonal allergies and have an increased tendency toward congestion and drooling due to the kapha predominance inherent to their life cycle. An increase in epileptic seizures and psychological disturbances during a full moon is another example of disease due to time cycles.

NATURAL DISORDERS: Imbalances that occur as a part of the normal dynamics of day-to-day life. Hunger, thirst, and feeling exhausted after exercise are not disorders, but temporary imbalances that require management through balanced lifestyle routines. Ayurveda generally considers these to be physiological expressions, but if you don't regulate them, they can progress and express as real disease as in the case of not eating when you feel hungry, which can lead to hyperacidity and gastritis.

NON-COMPREHENDIBLE DISORDERS: Imbalances that occur without known reasons or specific warnings. Burn or electric shock from lightning, injuries, and epidemics are some examples.

Ayurveda classifies the causative factors of disease in a wholly comprehensive manner. Etiological factors may be internal or external, but even the internal causative factors are generated or stimulated by external factors. For example, a disorder that occurs due to an innate hereditary defect, which would be considered an internal etiology, is usually triggered by external factors such as diet and lifestyle irregularities favorable to the manifestation of the ailment. Diabetes is an apt example, as it typically expresses due to extreme stressful internal or external conditions. External agents are not only physical in nature; impacts generated from the mind are also considered external to the system. For example, the death of a close relative occurs externally, but the grief and worry you experience in the face of crisis will affect your mind and body functions.

According to Ayurveda, there are three universal reasons for health and disease: improper use of sense organs, knowingly doing wrong things, and the impact of time cycles.

IMPROPER USE OF SENSES

As we've discussed, the five sense organs—eyes, nose, tongue, skin, and ears—are the portals that connect your child's inner self to the external world. These sense organs inform every perception children have of good/bad, pleasant/fearful, hot/cold, and every emotion they feel whether happiness, sadness, desire, aversion, generosity, greed, compassion, competition, pride, kindness, envy, and so on. When children use their senses in an improper way, all of their perceptions become distorted, and as a result, their entire mind-body systems' responses will also be distorted.

Think about the times your eyes play tricks on you and distort your view of something—perhaps while driving at night or sitting outside in the evening. Maybe you've seen the same effects in your children. When a young child sees a favorite teddy bear in the corner of a well-lit room, for example, they might go over and hug it, whereas if they see the same teddy bear in a dim light, they may become frightened and run away fearing there is something strange in the room. Imbalanced perceptions add to the formation or aggravation of diseases in children as well as adults.

ACTING AGAINST INTELLECT

If someone asked you whether you "knowingly do wrong things," your automatic response might be "no, of course not." But if you really analyze and observe your thoughts and the things you do throughout the day, you will see that on closer inspection it's likely a very different story.

Do you drink multiple cups of coffee a day despite knowing coffee isn't good for you and may even make you feel jittery and out of sorts? How about drinking ice water, eating at irregular times or while watching TV, or sleeping very late? You might find it an interesting exercise to make a list throughout a single day of the different ways you knowingly engage in actions you know are detrimental or unhealthy, and then think about how many of those routines you may unconsciously impose on your children. We all find excuses for doing what is pleasurable in the moment when we don't think the repercussions will be so bad. But when we consider how each small choice knocks our systems a little out of balance and the cumulative effect of these decisions day after day, we can see that the impact may be greater than we think. Ayurveda invites you to more consciously explore your own habits and behaviors so you can experience your own internal transformations and support your children in the most authentic way possible.

Ayurveda considers acting against intellect one of the main causes of disease. Making unhealthy choices despite an intellectual awareness of what is suitable or ideal encourages sensory temptations that overpower your intellect and take control of the mind. Any act committed regardless of intellect, willpower, or memory is considered an error if it causes an untoward result. Our intellects allow us to reason out the correct decision. Will or willpower is the mental strength to stay on a righteous path and steer away from incorrect deeds. And memory provides us with prior examples of actions and outcomes that let us know the particulars of better decision-making. A conscious, healthy individual initiates action only with proper application of all three.

With so many opportunities for full-grown, mature adults to make mistakes all day long, imagine how life feels for children with such young, vulnerable minds and hearts prone to constant temptation—their memory is short and their intellect and willpower as yet undeveloped. It is a parent's responsibility to understand this weakness and vulnerability and manage it in a positive way. As you can attest to, parents face all kinds of situations morning, noon, and night that give you the opportunity to encourage positive shifts within your children—even if that means sometimes following their temptations in a limited way to help them maintain emotional balance.

A lot of parents tend to reflexively say no a great deal of the time when their children ask to do one particular thing or another without offering any explanation. While they may have very clear reasons to deny these impulsive requests, they may not be aware of the impact this type of blunt refusal and denial can have on a child's mind. This type of response affects your child's entire mind-body system, and over time can cause them to become depressed or turn rebellious at home due to built-up frustration and discouragement. Dr. J has found that when children are very insistent on something—even when you think it's something you shouldn't allow—the more positive approach is to concede some quantity of what they desire and then explain the reasons why this isn't something you should do together very often.

For example, let's say your child has been asking to go for an ice cream after school and persists every day from the minute they see you that you take them to the ice cream shop. Instead of continuing to say no over and over, you could take them for a little treat, enjoy the moment with them, and then explain afterward the reasons it's not good for them to have ice cream before dinner very often. Spend time with your children in situations like this and let them know you hear how important their desires are to you. This will create an opportunity to talk lovingly with them about some healthier options for the future you can both agree on. This is mind care—keeping your children happy, peaceful, and feeling supported and positive, an aspect just as important as establishing healthy diet and lifestyle routines.

EFFECTS OF IMBALANCED TIME CYCLES

As we have discussed, variations in time cycles and rhythms can also lead to imbalances and impact internal physiological and emotional harmony. These include circadian rhythms, seasonal rhythms, and even the cycle of life. According to Ayurveda, even derangement of the seasons can trigger disease. Let's take a look at what this means. A season is considered "proper" when it carries its associated natural properties and intensity. For example, a proper summer has an optimal amount of light and heat expected for a particular geographical area. If a summer is too hot, it creates an excess with all living beings, and that excess heat leads to pitta aggravation. When a summer isn't as hot as it should be, this will have impacts of deficiency on the earth and cause dullness. In other cases, when a summer emits untoward radiation that extends into the fall, or winter cold extends into the spring season, for example, this will also have negative impacts on all living systems and beings.

Six Stages of Disease

Ayurveda identifies disease as a six-stage process and has the profound ability to recognize disease before it fully manifests, which makes it easier to prevent, treat, and cure.

Every disease process initiates with causative factors and emerges primarily from imbalances of the doshas. The causative factors are generally the elements that have increased a specific dosha or doshas and caused unwanted accumulation: the first stage. If the causative factors persist, the increased dosha is then carried into a further state of aggravation: the second stage of disease. In the third stage, the aggravated doshas begin to spread across the entire mind-body system. During the first three stages of disease, symptoms will generally be dosha-based and still easily treatable. When you identify imbalances prior to the fourth stage of disease, preventive protocols are usually all that are needed to effectively treat the disease.

In the fourth stage, the dosha or doshas that spread the imbalance in stage three localize in the body's weakest organs or systems and begin to alter function or physical structure—or sometimes both. Once localization occurs, disease enters the fifth stage of manifestation, when the cardinal signs and symptoms of the disease appear. If untreated, it can progress to the sixth stage of advanced disease and complication. Ayurveda considers the first three stages of disease in a preventative phase as the disease has not yet manifested whereas the last three stages require curative action.

Clinical presentation of disorders can be different in children than in adults despite similar dosha and organ involvement because the nature of an illness varies according to age. Ayurvedic assessment of children requires a comprehensive consultation that includes clinical observations, physical examination, diagnostic methodologies, and a detailed interview with the parents and children.

Ayurvedic Principle of Chikitsa

The main goal of Ayurvedic treatment, known as *chikitsa*, is to preserve, nurture, and nourish an individual's core vitality with the intention of not only curing the existing disease but also preventing further relapses or complications by bringing the mind-body system back to a normal, balanced state.

The primary difference between Ayurvedic medicine and modern medicine is where the focus lies. Ayurveda concentrates on managing the reasons for the imbalance that gave rise to the symptoms, whereas modern medicine fixates on immediate symptomatic relief. Parents often desire the same and identify disease with their child's symptoms and relief as an indication of healing. But symptoms are not disease; they are indicators of disease.

Let's take another look at childhood allergies: A child who suffers from breathlessness due to allergy-induced asthma may get sudden symptomatic relief from a bronchodilator, but over time the lungs will suffer greater exposure to the allergens that can lead to more complicated issues in the future. I am not suggesting a child be allowed to suffer with breathlessness! This is why Western medicine and Ayurveda can be complementary: modern medicine cares for the immediate acute symptoms while Ayurveda takes a longer view of the disease to provide a long-term, sustainable outcome. The Ayurvedic approach to this disorder would be to provide a complete protocol that enhances your child's immune resistance against allergens and strengthens the lungs, which in turn will help relieve symptoms along with the bronchodilator.

You may find it interesting that Ayurveda considers digestion and metabolism (agni) the most important factors in healing an individual from any disease. The reason for this is that agni is responsible for all of the biotransformations within the body. Since balanced digestion and metabolism are criteria to sustain optimal health, that is Ayurveda's first and primary goal when managing disease. Once a person's agni is addressed, priority is given to balancing the dosha or doshas involved in the disease process. Next comes the repair and rejuvenation of the organ or system involved in the disease. Finally, we work toward relieving the presentations or symptoms. This stepwise process doesn't mean waiting for agni to be completely corrected before addressing the real pathology or symptoms. Appropriate measures are taken concurrently to pacify the involved doshas, which in turn begin to work on the affected organ or system, and the individual components slowly, collectively come back into balance. At the same time, various steps are taken to alleviate a person's symptoms and establish a complete treatment protocol that includes following healthy lifestyle habits and a specified diet regimen.

When you follow these principles with the guidance of an Ayurvedic physician, it not only alleviates the disease, but eradicates the causes that manifested the illness. At the same time, various steps are taken to alleviate a person's symptoms and establish a complete treatment protocol that may include some of the traditional Ayurvedic therapies you'll find below along with following healthy lifestyle habits to balance the doshas assessed by the nature of the disease or disorder.

Traditional Ayurvedic Therapies

There are many bodywork techniques mentioned in the ancient texts that are commonly used as stand-alone procedures and as components of therapeutic interventions. These Ayurvedic therapies can be beneficial for maintaining health and used as treatment modalities for specific disorders. Ayurveda considers skin one of the most important routes of therapeutic administration, and an experienced Ayurvedic physician will be able to select therapies as well as the best oils or ingredients for each procedure for a wholly tailored and unique healing treatment. There are many such therapies commonly used in the management of both physical and mental childhood disorders: let's look at some of the main ones.

ABHYANGA

According to the ancient texts of Ayurveda, *abhyanga,* or whole-body oil massage, is indicated as a daily application to prevent dryness and the process of degeneration. This therapy supports the body physically, mentally, and emotionally while balancing the doshas. Its rhythmic motion helps to relieve stiffness from the joints and muscles and free body movements. This stimulating treatment increases blood circulation, which in turn encourages quick removal of metabolic wastes while at the same time providing relief for conditions such as anxiety, fatigue, circulatory disorders, and dryness. Abhyanga enables sound sleep, increases one's general sense of well-being and life span, and also improves the complexion and texture of the skin.

SHASHTIKA LEPA

A traditional body massage administered with cooked Njavara rice after liberal application of medicated oil over the entire body is known as *shashtika lepa.* Njavara is a variety of red rice known to be highly nourishing and strengthening. It is cooked into a soft paste in cow's milk then mixed with an herbal decoction. The paste is applied all over the body to induce sudation (sweat). This procedure is highly rejuvenating, nourishing, and prepares the individual to bear the stress and strain of a busy lifestyle. It enhances physical consistency, strengthens the nervous system, and improves the overall appearance of the skin.

SHIROLEPA

In this procedure, an herbal paste is applied externally to the scalp. For children with an intellectual disability or other cognitive issues, the paste is made from a combination of licorice, Indian gooseberry, and *musta* (nut grass). *Shirolepa* is also effective in the management of psoriasis, dandruff, and scalp lesions.

KARNA POORANA

Karna poorana is an ancient Ayurvedic healing therapy for ear ailments using lukewarm herbal or medicated Ayurvedic oils. This Ayurvedic therapy offers effective relief to patients suffering from earaches and certain conditions of the head and neck, including pain.

NASYA

Nasya is a traditional Ayurvedic therapy for the nose, throat, sinuses, and head. The face, shoulders, and chest are massaged with specific herbal oils to cause therapeutic perspiration. The herbal oil is measured in an exact dose and instilled into the nostrils so the individual can slowly inhale it. This Ayurvedic therapy is known to prevent allergies, sinusitis, headaches, migraine, rhinitis, and other nasal issues. Therapeutic oils for nasya need to be selected by an Ayurvedic professional based on the individual and disease tendencies. This therapy will cleanse, purify, and strengthen the nasal passages to breathe fully and easily again.

PICHU

A thick layer of cotton wool or a gauze pad soaked with a warm herbal oil is applied over affected areas and changed periodically in a warming cycle. *Pichu* therapy is used in children with ADHD, autism, and other cognitional issues utilizing specific traditional oils. It is also effective for degenerative and painful problems like back pain and for healing injuries.

Shirodhara is a traditional Ayurvedic therapy that involves pouring medicated liquid, usually oils, over the forehead with a rhythmic side-to-side oscillation for a stipulated period of time. The rhythm of these oscillations is of much importance as it stimulates the seat of our cognition, which results in channelization of bio-energies and restoration of good health. Shirodhara rejuvenates and revitalizes body and mind and ultimately strengthens the physical constitution of the individual. It relieves stress and strain-related problems, imparts better vision and hearing, and clears several nasal problems.

In *shirovasti*, specially prepared warm medicated oil is poured inside a tall leakproof cap, attached firmly around the head, and sealed with black lentil paste. The oil is kept lukewarm throughout the process. Shirovasti is traditionally done for vata conditions such as headaches, ear diseases, degenerative brain disorders, cerebral palsy, lesions of the brain, epilepsy, and others.

o o o

Diabetes is now one of the most common metabolic disorders around the globe. Identifying increased sugar levels in the blood is the simplest method to confirm diabetes. Based on Ayurvedic teachings, diabetes falls under a group of conditions termed *prameha*, expressed as excessive and altered manifestations of urine and comprised of twenty different stages. If the initial stages of prameha are untreated, it can develop into *madhumeha*, increased sugar levels in the blood and urine with excessive urination. An expert Ayurvedic doctor can identify tendencies headed toward diabetes in a patient long before they reach the stage of increased sugar in the blood and urine. The ability to pinpoint these disease tendencies before manifestation is unique to the science of Ayurvedic medicine.

o   o   o

Many parents and caregivers unnecessarily turn to over-the-counter medications because they don't want to see their children suffering. While the intent is justifiable from an emotional perspective, such practices not only mask your child's symptoms but also give the underlying disease a chance to progress or even create irreversible complications from undesirable side effects of OTC drugs.

Dr. J remembers one pediatric case in India when a child suffered from a ruptured appendix followed by severe post-surgery complications of intestinal adhesions. When the child mentioned to his parents that his stomach pain had become unbearable, they thought it was from running around and playing with his friends and began giving him over-the-counter painkillers. They continued this regimen every day for a week and thought he was getting better since the pain had subsided—only it hadn't. The pills were just masking the symptoms of a serious underlying condition, and no one had any idea until the boy collapsed and was taken to a nearby hospital. As this story illustrates, in most cases, symptoms are *indicators* of disease that will point you toward the root of the problem. Masking symptoms can lead to progression of underlying disease and complications.

When you tune in to the underlying causes of your child's complaints on a day-to-day basis, you'll often find that natural home remedies and treatments can work wonders—without any unwanted side effects. For example, colicky pain after a meal with feelings of heaviness in the stomach indicates indigestion. What would be the point in giving your child medicine in that case? You could instead prepare a simple tea with cumin seed and a bit of ginger and ask your child to refrain from eating anything for a few hours while their symptoms slowly disappear.

Ayurvedic healing starts with uncovering and avoiding the cause of disorder followed by remedying the core underlying imbalances that create disharmony in the mind and body systems. In the next chapters, we will discuss the Ayurvedic perspective on specific childhood health conditions along with principles of prevention and management.

13

MIND-RELATED DISORDERS

CHILDREN TODAY ARE often more stressed than parents and suffering from mental, behavioral, and developmental health conditions that affect a person's thinking, feeling, behavior, and moods. An estimated 50 percent of all lifetime mental health disorders begin by the age of fourteen. The question on so many parents' minds today—especially if you have a child yourself diagnosed with a mental health issue—is *Why?* Why are these diagnoses increasing at such an alarming rate, and why are so many children in distress? There are many underlying factors for disease according to the science of Ayurveda, which we will discuss throughout this chapter, but common denominators of unhealthy behaviors and chronic childhood disorders are lifestyle, environment, and stress.

Whereas modern medicine views most mental health issues in children as entirely brain-related, Ayurveda identifies certain aspects of the mind that work not only with the brain but also independent of the brain. While intellectual, analytical, and factual memory are connected to brain function, Ayurveda correlates emotional aspects of the mind such as unconditional love, empathy, and compassion to the heart. Due to this wide scope and understanding of the mind, the science of Ayurveda adopts multifaceted treatment methodologies that influence the brain as well as the aspects of the mind that are not controlled by the brain. *Satvavajaya Chikitsa* (Ayurvedic psychotherapy) is a nonpharmacological method aimed at controlling the mind and restraining it from unwholesome objects (*ahita artha*), or stressors.

Mental disorders in children are usually first identified when parents and caregivers observe major changes in the ways children typically behave, learn, and cope with their emotions, which often lead to greater distress and challenges throughout the day. It's common, of course, for healthy children to feel irritable, sad, or fearful at times and occasionally experience difficulties staying focused, but severe changes in behavior that persist over time and affect school activities, social life, and behavior at home are indications of a mental disorder.

When your child's mind is balanced, they reach social-emotional and developmental milestones and acquire meaningful skills that allow them to play happily with friends, cooperate, help others, and effectively cope with feelings and behavior. A healthy mind reflects a happy, enthusiastic child at school, home, and in their community.

Ayurveda's approach to children's mental health is not limited to managing a diagnosis but includes treatment therapies aimed at improving and enhancing abilities related to perception, analysis, decision-making, and memory so they can respond to life with a positive attitude and balanced state of mind. The most common mind-related disorders in children are ADHD, autism spectrum disorder, developmental delays, anxiety, bed-wetting, and night terrors. Let's consider Ayurveda's perspective on these conditions.

ADHD

ADHD is one of the most diagnosed neurodevelopmental childhood disorders in the modern world. Fundamentally, children are prone to such disorders during this stage of life because of the young, delicate nature of their heart and mind. The possible etiological factors for children diagnosed with ADHD are many and can stem from both genetic and environmental influences before and after birth. These include undernourishment of the fetus, premature delivery, imbalances during pregnancy (dietary, lifestyle, mental and emotional, alcohol or tobacco use), poor nutrition, and exposure to toxic chemicals.

According to Ayurveda, ADHD is a vata disorder of the mind often associated with pitta. Symptoms of ADHD primarily indicate a vata aggravation and express in many different ways including increased restlessness, emotional instability, tics and fidgeting, excessive talking, daydreaming, increased forgetfulness, and carelessness. From the Ayurvedic perspective, there also exists an exaggeration of symptoms during the last phase of digestion and a tendency to have low body weight. In cases with a pitta association there can be increased anger, aggression, and a tendency for self-harm.

In a climate of increasing ADHD assessments and diagnosis rates in children and adolescents, many parents and caregivers have obvious concerns about potential for overdiagnosis and the long-term effects of treatment. Misdiagnosis is a controversial subject in today's culture. In Dr. J's experience, children can be diagnosed with ADHD who have tendencies to be only slightly more active than other children in their age group without any major behavioral issues. This is a limitation of the current system that uses incomplete and subjective diagnostic criteria to assess and define mind function. Ayurveda views the mind as profoundly complex in nature, and while it doesn't have a physical existence, it controls all of the sensory perceptions and responses to stimuli.

Ayurvedic management of ADHD is very comprehensive and considers every aspect of a child's mind, body, and environment. Since it is a vata-predominant condition with pitta association, the overall treatment principle/protocol is to nourish, stabilize, and strengthen the mind-body systems, especially the brain and mind. While regular psychosocial interventions and behavioral therapies such as speech therapy and occupational therapy are immensely helpful for children to learn tools for managing their day-to-day life, healing and recovery from ADHD also requires dietary, lifestyle, and therapeutic interventions.

In addition to following the basic principles of Ayurvedic nutrition we discussed in chapter 4 such as establishing regular mealtimes and avoiding cold food and beverages, it is especially important to provide your child food and ingredients known to pacify both vata and pitta with the ability to nourish and strengthen the nervous system and mind. Some examples include cultured ghee, winter melon, cultured butter, black raisins, red rice, coconut, Indian gooseberry, and pomegranate.

As you have learned, your child's lifestyle practices are essential to correcting imbalances and maintaining good health. The best way you can support your child is by helping them follow a regular daily routine that includes a moderate level of physical activity, going to bed early, limiting screen time, and spending time relaxing in a family environment. There's no need to be overly regimented or strict; life is meant to be enjoyable and carefree—just do your best not to let unhealthy habits creep in too often!

Specific practices Ayurveda recommends for managing ADHD include daily, full-body oil application (abhyanga), or body massage (refer to chapter 16 for oil suggestions), warm showers, and application of sandalwood paste at the center of the forehead between the eyebrows in cases of pitta association. Making time for slow and steady deep breathing sessions as part of a fun family activity and playing calming, stabilizing mantras for your children will create a soothing, grounding home environment.

The basic therapeutic regimen an Ayurvedic physician will undertake includes clearing the mind-body channels, pacifying vata and pitta, undergoing a mild purification if necessary to eliminate aggravated doshas and accumulated toxins from the body, followed by the final stage of rejuvenation therapy (rasayana) that uses traditional herbs and Ayurvedic formulations such as Brahmi Ghrita and Kalyanaka Ghrita to rejuvenate the mind and nervous system. Rasayana, or rejuvenation therapy, deeply nourishes and strengthens the body to prevent recurrences of disorders and provide a sustained clinical outcome to the Ayurvedic healing regimen. Traditional Ayurvedic body therapies such as abhyanga, shirolepa, shashtika lepa, shirovasti, nasya, and pichu can also be highly effective performed under the supervision of an Ayurvedic doctor.

Since the causes of ADHD are commonly linked to genetic factors, derangements that occur during the fetal period, and labor complications, the best thing parents can do when they are planning to have a child is to prepare for a healthy pregnancy.

Traditional Ayurvedic preconception care starts with both parents having a complete Ayurvedic assessment and receiving guidance on lifestyle routines based on constitution and present health status. Many couples and individuals preparing for pregnancy choose to embark on a complete physical and spiritual journey during the preconception period that includes an Ayurvedic cleanse (panchakarma) followed by rejuvenation practices (rasayana) to optimize all aspects of fertility and conception through the Ayurvedic lens. Taking these steps can minimize the possibility of your child developing ADHD and help prevent pregnancy complications.

EPIGENETICS

All too often, the accepted way of thinking cements ideas that there is nothing you can do about genetic tendencies and hereditary disorders. The science of Ayurveda rejects this belief and completely aligns with the emerging principles of epigenetics that recognize we have the outright ability to downregulate our own disease tendencies as well as upregulate epigenetic patterns that can cause changes to affect the way our genes work. Epigenetics is an emerging field, and literally means "above" or "on top of" genetics. The preventive and curative guidelines of Ayurveda rest entirely on our capability to resist disease and degeneration through diet, lifestyle, mind care practices, natural healing ingredients, detoxification, and rejuvenation protocols. Our genes play an important role in our health, but so do our behaviors, environment, and lifestyles. According to the CDC, "While *genetic* changes can alter which protein is made, *epigenetic* changes affect gene expression to turn genes 'on' and 'off.' Since your environment and behaviors, such as diet and exercise, can result in epigenetic changes, it is easy to see the connection between your genes and your behaviors and environment."[1]

Autism Spectrum Disorder

Autism spectrum disorder (ASD) covers a range of developmental debility causing significant challenges and limitations in behavior, social skills, and communication. A distinctive feature of this condition is that children with ASD present a wide array of behavioral patterns with varying degrees of severity. There are gifted ASD children with superior cognitive skills and various exceptional abilities that exceed what most other children demonstrate. At the same time, some ASD children face severe challenges and need a lot of support in their daily lives. In most cases, growth and physical development of children with ASD are equal to typical norms for children, but differences in the way their brains develop affect the ways they learn, behave, and communicate.

The causative factors are similar to ADHD and include genetic disorders, environmental factors, and maternal lifestyle imbalances and disease during pregnancy (depression, addiction, stress, depression, and emotional trauma). The signs of ASD usually start during early childhood and typically express with unusual and repetitive movements and behaviors. Other common symptoms include unresponsiveness, trouble making eye contact, not showing interest in other people, an inability to recognize emotions or have empathy, reluctance to be touched or to cuddle, repeating or echoing words or phrases, difficulty expressing needs, and becoming easily frustrated. Ayurveda classifies ASD as a vata-predominant condition with the association of other doshas in some cases.

Early systematic psychosocial interventions and behavioral therapies focused on social communication development and reduction of repetitive behavior are essential tools that can help minimize symptoms profoundly and help children transition into the mainstream as they get older. Ayurveda recommends following a balanced Ayurvedic diet guided by the healthy eating principles we have discussed along with increasing foods known to pacify vata and strengthen the mind and nervous system. Modifying your child's lifestyle habits is key to supporting any Ayurvedic regimen and should include going to bed early, regular physical activity, and a limited amount of screen exposure. Regular full-body oil application and massage also supports vata pacification. Ayurvedic therapeutic protocols need to be customized based on your child's prakriti, age, and stage of ASD as guided by an Ayurvedic doctor. The overall treatment principle is to pacify vata and provide Ayurvedic herbs that strengthen and rejuvenate the mind and nervous system such as *shankhapushpi*, brahmi, and madukaparni. Ayurvedic bodywork techniques including abhyanga, shirodhara, shirolepa, and pichu are found to be very effective in calming and stabilizing the unique body-mind systems of affected children. Listening to mantra chanting on a regular basis can be calming and emotionally stabilizing for children with ASD.

As with ADHD, the causes of ASD are mostly related to genetic factors and complications during pregnancy and the perinatal period. As mentioned earlier, Ayurvedic preconception care is a profound traditional protocol guided by an Ayurvedic physician that goes beyond prenatal medical screening tests and offers couples and women planning a pregnancy a comprehensive path to prepare the mind and body for a healthy pregnancy. This unique health care program integrates counseling on conscious conception with a systematic orientation that prepares the womb for balanced fetal development and supports mental and emotional preparedness for this profound journey.

Developmental Delays

Children unable to stand or walk on their own by the age of one indicate developmental delays and conditions known collectively as *phakka* in Ayurveda. These delays can occur in many areas and may affect cognition, communication, speech, and motor skills as well as social, emotional, and behavioral skills. Cognitive delays interfere with awareness and influence learning abilities, intellectual functions, communication, and interaction with others. Often, children present with delays in more than one area of development, known as global developmental delay.

Etiologies of developmental delays in children range from a variety of prenatal, perinatal, and postnatal factors to socioeconomic and environmental causes that can impact a child's growth and development. The ancient Ayurvedic texts classify causes of developmental delays in children into three primary types: impairment of intrauterine, embryonic, and fetal nourishment that affects the development of a child, or *garbhaja phakka*; deficiencies in the quality and quantity of breast milk that can lead to diminished and delayed growth and mental development in children, or *ksheeraja phakka*; and chronic diseases such as recurrent abdominal and respiratory infections, intestinal parasites, bleeding disorders, and metabolic and endocrine diseases during the neonatal period that decelerate the growth and overall development of a child, or *vyadhija phakka*.

Ayurvedic management of developmental delays begins with assessing and managing underlying disease such as gut infections or intestinal parasites known to put children at high risk for growth delays. The second step is supporting digestion and absorption of nutrients by correcting agni along with gut dynamics like grahani. The incorporation of simple digestive spices, consuming food at the correct time, and preparing easily digestible and nourishing meals are common guidelines parents can follow. External application of traditional Ayurvedic oils known to enhance nourishment and strength is also recommended at home, and these can be found in chapter 16.

Ayurveda offers many traditional herbs known to enhance digestive strength and nourish all of the body systems along with specific therapeutic formulations to rejuvenate the mind. These can help parents manage speech and cognitive delays. An experienced Ayurvedic physician will create a treatment plan for your child that customizes herbal remedies along with therapies that include shashtika lepa, shirolepa, shiro pichu, and abhyanga for a complete treatment protocol.

Anxiety

Anxiety can be seen across different stages of a child's development and affects many children of all different ages: toddlers throw tantrums, elementary school children refuse to get dressed on the first day of school, and teenagers experience heart palpitations and other symptoms when studying for an upcoming exam, for example. Since younger children especially aren't always able to articulate their feelings to their parents, anxiety expresses through temper tantrums, excessive screaming, crying, misbehavior, difficulty sleeping, and nightmares. Although some of these feelings and experiences are part of everyday life and considered typical, generalized anxiety is quite common among children—and on the rise. If your child repeatedly worries about matters before they happen or has constant concerns about school, sports, or friends, it can affect normal childhood activities. Other signs of anxiety include intense fear and phobias and a wide range of physical symptoms such as headaches, nausea, shortness of breath, stomachache, tremors, and digestive issues. Anxiety medications are widely prescribed to children today to help manage their anxiety and day-to-day activities.

Ayurveda understands childhood anxiety as a vata-predominant condition. Known causes of anxiety disorders include hereditary and congenital factors as well as negative exposures and childhood traumas. It is the delicate nature of a child's mind that makes them vulnerable to anxiety and mental disorders. Traditional Ayurvedic herbs and formulations that support rejuvenation of the mind (*medhya rasayana*) including shankhapushpi, brahmi, and yashtimadhu combined with herbal adaptogens such as ashwagandha are especially beneficial. These should be prescribed by an Ayurvedic professional.

Lifestyle routines are key in helping children manage anxiety and provide many opportunities to establish a healthy way of living and restore balance to a child's mind. Ayurveda recommends parents make every effort to follow a warm, unctuous, vata-pacifying diet that favors sweet, sour, and salty tastes and do their best to adhere to regular sleep times. Oleation or abhyanga is very soothing and effective for relieving anxiety and can be incorporated into your child's daily routine along with other lifestyle therapies such as listening to soothing mantras playing softly in the bedroom and adopting yoga practices that include deep belly breathing, Yoga Nidra, and balancing yoga sequences with plenty of seated postures. You can wind down these practices with a simple guided meditation at bedtime, for example, or whenever you notice your child needs to relax. Remember, keeping these activities light, fun, and part of a regular routine will help achieve the best outcome for your child.

Bed-Wetting

Bed-wetting, or nocturnal enuresis, is the condition of involuntary urination at night after five years of age and can be due to both physiological and psychological etiologies. Causes include small bladder capacity, lack of bladder control, and hormonal issues along with anxiety, stress, and developmental disorders issues like ASD. Bed-wetting can have emotional impacts on both the affected children and their family members. The most important thing for parents to be aware of is that bed-wetting is neither their child's fault nor under their control. Some common management techniques include counseling for parents, bladder training, conditioning therapy, regulation of water intake in the evening, and ensuring a child voids their bladder just before going to bed.

From the Ayurvedic perspective, this is a vitiated vata condition, specific to the aspect of vata that controls downward movements including elimination (*apana vata*). Ayurveda recommends vata pacifying and strengthening herbs and rejuvenating formulations specific to the mind. Most children overcome bed-wetting with suggested supports, but in cases where there isn't noted improvement with such modifications, more extensive clinical investigations may be required to identify possible neurological abnormalities.

Night Terrors and Nightmares

Night terrors and nightmares are common childhood conditions that occur in different stages of the sleep cycle. All children cycle through light sleep or rapid eye movement (REM) and deep sleep or non-rapid eye movement (NREM) throughout the night. After falling into a deep stage of sleep, children typically stay in that stage for the first few hours of the night and then alternate between deep and light sleep. Night terrors generally occur prior to midnight when children get "stuck" between the deep and light sleep stages. Their body is "awake" but their mind is not, which causes a sudden onset of screaming with their eyes either open or closed, rapid breathing, and a fast heartbeat. They may look intensely afraid and can even run around shouting and screaming, which can be terrifying for parents. Usually, children won't remember anything in the morning because they have no awareness of what is happening during these episodes.

Nightmares usually occur after midnight during the dream stage of sleep, and children often wake in the middle of the night with extreme fear. Parents should comfort and hold their children until they feel relaxed and can return to bed. Frequent nightmares associated with symptoms such as recurrent headaches or variation in hunger levels can be an indication of underlying issues like bullying, academic problems, or family issues.

Since night terrors and nightmares occur at distinct times on different conscious levels, management approaches vary. Though it may seem counterintuitive, you should never try to wake or comfort your child during a night terror. This can further aggravate them and wake them completely, leaving the child very confused and making it difficult to go back to sleep. Parents should make sure their child is safe and stay nearby until the night terror subsides.

Fear is considered an expression of vata dosha. The best way to support children suffering from recurrent nightmares or night terrors is to follow a vata-pacifying diet and lifestyle. Daily routines should include a regular pranayama practice of slow and steady Alternate Nostril Breathing, simple meditation sessions, and massage with vata-pacifying oils. Parents can also apply a few drops of soothing, calming Ayurvedic oil to the crown of their child's head before bedtime to help calm the mind and nervous system and promote a restful night's sleep. Spending time with your children having positive, reassuring conversations can be very supportive in helping them overcome these tendencies.

Ayurvedic herbs including brahmi, guduchi, shankhapushpi, and *mandukaparni* are known for their calming and rejuvenating effects on the mind (*medhya rasyana*) and may be suggested by an Ayurvedic physician along with bodywork techniques and oil therapies.

There are many other mind-related disorders that affect children, and this is by no means a complete list, but rather a sample of common examples of mind-related disorders in children to describe the Ayurvedic approach to healing the mind. You can understand treatment of other mind-related conditions the same way as Ayurveda corrects all possible disorders within one system based on the same management principles. Above all, your dedicated and loving mental and emotional support along with creating and maintaining balanced lifestyle routines for your children can support healing all types of mind-related conditions.

14

DIGESTIVE AND METABOLIC DISORDERS

AYURVEDA CONSIDERS THE digestive system the "master system" of the body. The digestive system is the main port of entry for ingesting the food required to nourish every system in the body. The entire process of digestion including nourishment of tissues as well as available energy depends on the health of the digestive system. It is not only what we eat but the strength and balance of the digestive system and agni that determine whether the entire mind-body system gets nourished.

Ayurveda assesses digestive health by the state of a person's agni. Imbalances of the digestive fire are considered the main cause of various diseases of the digestive system including those of the esophagus, stomach, small intestine, and colon. Therefore, kindling agni and reestablishing its capacity to digest food properly is the main treatment principle in managing disorders of the digestive system.

Ayurveda always discusses the concept of metabolism in terms of digestion. In Ayurvedic terms, metabolism refers to subtle digestion, when absorbed nutrients in the gut are further transformed into the various tissues, energies, and vitality after gross digestion from ingestion to absorption in the intestinal tract. Since subtle digestion occurs in all of the tissues and organs, it is also called cellular digestion. The nutrients from the gut are transformed into energy and absorbed by the body's various tissues in the process of metabolism that occurs at a cellular level. Therefore, metabolic disorders are also considered a derangement of the body's subtle agni, which includes hormones and other factors of cellular metabolism. Correcting this imbalance is Ayurveda's primary focus.

Impairments of digestive strength and metabolism can affect a child's growth and development and sometimes lead to lifelong issues such as asthma, cardiovascular disease, and high blood pressure. Ayurveda's approach to pediatric health management is always to maintain a child's healthy digestion by sustaining balanced agni. Some of the most common digestive conditions that affect children today are stomachache, indigestion, vomiting, and diarrhea along with the metabolic disorders of obesity and diabetes. Let's look at the Ayurvedic approach to managing these conditions.

Stomachache and Indigestion

Tummy trouble tops the list of common issues for children, but their complaints can sometimes be difficult for parents to interpret because the pain is often nonspecific. In many cases, the location of pain in the abdomen along with the nature of the pain can help identify the issue.

Typically, when your child gets a stomachache after eating, it is usually due to indigestion. Burning sensations in the upper abdomen accompanied by acid reflux and sour belching are signs of hyperacidity and inflammation of the stomach lining, commonly known as gastritis. Lower abdominal pain and spasms followed by diarrhea are typically due to acute or chronic conditions in the colon such as dysentery or IBS and usually subside in a few hours or days depending on the nature of the condition. However, if your child complains about a stomachache that won't go away or recurrent abdominal pain, it's important to call your child's physician for an assessment. Prompt medical care avoids unnecessary complications. Anytime you're unsure if your child's symptoms warrant a visit to the doctor, it's always best to call your pediatrician.

The most common reasons for indigestion and stomachache in children are:

- Overeating
- Eating before the previous meal is completely digested
- Eating foods that are hard to digest like oily and fried foods, cheese, and too many raw salads or vegetables
- Eating uncooked or half-cooked food
- Eating excessively sweet, sour, and salty food
- Sleeping immediately after meals
- Drinking lots of water during a meal

Ayurveda offers many natural and effective home remedies to ease spasms of the gut due to indigestion that may lead to colicky-type abdominal pain and cramps and recommends warm application both internally and externally to relieve pain. First and foremost, be aware that feeding your children cold or uncooked, raw foods anytime they have an upset stomach will increase their pain and discomfort. Prepare freshly cooked meals whenever possible and offer warm, easily digestible foods when your child feels hungry. When the digestive fire or agni runs low—which is often the case with indigestion and stomach pain—it's time to find some kindling! Think of your child's agni as a little campfire that has been extinguished or isn't burning brightly enough to fully cook or digest their food. Ayurveda offers various routines and recipes to rekindle and strengthen agni that you can find in chapter 5. Many of them start in the kitchen!

One of the best ways you can stoke your child's digestive fire is by using digestion-enhancing spices. A pinch of cumin, ginger, cardamom seed, or fennel seed in a cup of tea or bowl of soup, for example, is very beneficial for increasing agni and alleviating stomach pain and discomfort due to indigestion. Avoid cold, oily, or hard to digest foods that will dampen or extinguish agni until your child feels better and expresses a more regular pattern of hunger—a sure sign their digestive fire is burning brightly once again.

Another way you can use Ayurvedic herbs and spices is to transform certain foods and beverages into a more easily digestible form. Dairy is a great example. The usual practice, especially in the Western world, is to give children a glass of cold milk directly from the refrigerator. You can avoid indigestion and stomachaches and make the milk easier for your child to digest by diluting it first with some water and warming it up on the stove with a pinch of turmeric or ginger powder.

A simple and traditional Ayurvedic practice that uses external application of warmth to relieve colicky abdominal pain in children is to apply warm castor oil on the abdomen. You can heat it to lukewarm either on the stove or simply by rubbing it between your palms using friction. The application should be very light and ideally in a clockwise direction for a minute or so. Ayurveda recommends you press the pause button on all sports, exercise, and strenuous activities and encourage your child to rest until stomach pain fully resolves.

Vomiting and Diarrhea

Vomiting and diarrhea are common childhood conditions that can either signal a problem on their own or be symptoms of other illnesses like inflammatory bowel disorders or appendicitis. While vomiting or emesis is the forceful expulsion of stomach contents from the mouth, diarrhea expresses as frequent watery or loose stools. Vomiting is often associated with nausea, which can be a strange uneasy feeling for children. These conditions can affect your children's moods and behaviors, and sometimes make them anxious or even cry. Or they may become very quiet and subdued when they feel like they might throw up. Usually, they will want to lie down or go to bed early. Keeping your children company when they are under the weather helps them feel supported and protected and may even help speed up their recovery!

There are many causes of vomiting and diarrhea such as viruses, bacteria, food poisoning, indigestion, hyperacidity, gut inflammations, intestinal parasites, overeating, underlying medical conditions, or eating undercooked food. Ayurveda's primary consideration for both these conditions whether they occur on their own or together is the gut responding to something that it doesn't agree with, creating crisis for its normal function.

There can also be mental or emotional causes of vomiting such as stress or seeing something that creates aversions or disgusting feelings in the mind such as a pool of blood or an open wound or exposure to a foul smell, for example. Other disorders that cause vomiting are migraine headaches, motion sickness, imbalances of the inner ear like Ménière's disease, and behavioral issues like bulimia. The most common reasons for diarrhea in children are stomach infections like gastroenteritis, indigestion, and food intolerances and allergies to ingredients like gluten and dairy.

Vomiting and diarrhea are natural, protective urges your body expresses to expel harmful contents and should never be suppressed—especially in cases of toxicity, indigestion, or food poisoning. The general principles Ayurveda suggests you follow are to allow the body to purge whatever it needs to remove from the system and then support the body to avoid possible complications like dehydration and exhaustion. Cases with no substance to be expelled, such as overstimulation of the gastric or esophageal mucosa or excessive vagal stimulation, can affect nutrition and cause considerable discomfort, which needs to be either managed or treated depending on the root cause.

The most important advice to parents when your child vomits is to stay calm. Vomiting is frightening and exhausting to children, and if they see you worry or panic, they will be much more affected mentally by the episode. Reassuring your child and avoiding dehydration are key at this stage. A lot of parents make the mistake of feeding their child immediately after vomiting, thinking they are probably starving because the last meal is now out of their system. The fact is when you feed your child or encourage them to drink a lot of fluids at this point, it might cause the vomiting to continue. Resuming a normal diet when your child has diarrhea can also prolong the problem. The best practice is to wait to feed your child until the vomiting and diarrhea completely subside and sip fluids that can give your child some immediate energy as well as electrolyte balance. Prolonged bouts of these conditions can lead to dehydration, which can be serious if left untreated. Always watch for these signs of dehydration:

- Dry lips, dry mouth, and sometimes cracked lips
- Dry or wrinkled skin (notably on the abdomen and upper arms or legs)
- Absence of urination for 6–8 hours
- Reduced alertness or inactivity
- Weak, fast pulse
- Excessive sleepiness or disorientation
- Rapid and deep breathing with sunken eyes

Ayurveda identifies many simple kitchen ingredients and spices that can treat nausea, vomiting, and diarrhea in children. Fresh lime juice, cardamom, ginger, black pepper, and cumin can all relieve and soothe nausea and help stop vomiting. Sipping a tea made by boiling water with the skin of pomegranate fruit or a pinch of nutmeg powder with honey may help ease diarrhea. Here are some traditional Ayurvedic home remedies that can help you support your children's recovery:

- Add a teaspoon of lime juice to a cup of water at room temperature and blend with a teaspoon of unrefined cane sugar and a pinch of salt. Sipping this every few minutes can help soothe nausea, vomiting, and dehydration due to diarrhea.
- Boil a tablespoon of powdered puffed rice in a cup of water, add a teaspoon of unrefined cane sugar, and take 1 teaspoon of this mixture every ten to fifteen minutes to ease nausea and manage dehydration and exhaustion.
- Chewing one or two cardamom seeds can also help ease nausea.
- If the nausea, vomiting, and diarrhea are due to indigestion or the previous meal not agreeing with the stomach, mixing a few drops of ginger juice with a teaspoon of lemon juice and taking a few drops every few minutes can settle the stomach.
- Boiling ½ teaspoon of cumin seeds in a cup of water with a pinch of nutmeg, and sip frequently.
- Offer your child ½ teaspoon of equal parts natural raw honey and fresh lemon juice—another effective home remedy!

Obesity

According to Ayurveda, all diseases can be broadly classified into two categories: diseases due to overnutrition or accumulation (*santarpanaja roga*) and diseases due to depletion and degeneration (*apatarpanaja roga*). When material and energy inputs to the body exceed its normal outputs, accumulation and weight gain occur. On the contrary, when energy output is greater than energy input, this results in weight loss. In other words, metabolic diseases are either due to anabolic excess or catabolic excess; obesity is the former.

Obesity is a continuing epidemic in the United States and affects one in five children and adolescents. According to the National Center for Health Statistics (NCHS), 19.3 percent of children and adolescents ages two to nineteen are obese, affecting about 14.4 million individuals.[1] This serious, chronic disorder impacts every aspect of a child's life and also puts tremendous strain on families. Childhood obesity gives children and adolescents a much greater risk for poor health. Obesity is linked to many disorders including type 2 diabetes, heart disease, joint disorders, and cancers.

Body mass index (BMI) is commonly used to assess childhood weight status. It is calculated by dividing a person's weight in kilograms by the square of their height in meters. For children and adolescents, BMI is age- and gender-specific and varies based on these factors. Because of this, a child's BMI needs to be identified relative to other children of the same age group and gender. When a child's BMI is greater than the ninety-fifth percentile, they would be considered obese.

Ayurveda identifies obesity as a kapha-predominant disorder. While there are many potential causes of childhood obesity, these are considered the most common:

- Overeating and having meals too frequently
- Excessive fried, sweet, and fatty foods
- Lack of exercise or sedentary lifestyle
- Excessive sleeping, especially during the daytime
- Hereditary factors

- Increased stress and emotional disturbances
- Derangement of agni that includes subtle hormonal imbalances

Ayurveda considers obesity a major disease (*maha roga*), meaning a complex condition that affects multiple body systems and can be difficult to manage. Due to one or more of these causes, the digestive and metabolic fire (agni) can weaken and affect the transformation of food and nutrients to energy for various tissues, causing an accumulation of fat in the body. Since this process slows down the efficient processing of energy, these children often experience a decrease in energy levels and feelings of laziness that in turn make them more sedentary and causes further accumulation.

The key factor that makes obesity such a difficult condition to manage is that it increases hunger. Let's take a look at how that happens. You probably know that fat is an insulator. The increased development of the body's layers of fat makes it difficult for heat to dissipate from the inner body. When that heat accumulates inside the body, it expresses as increased hunger. As a child's hunger increases beyond normal levels, there will be a tendency to eat larger quantities of food more frequently. And here's where things become even more complicated. The stress mechanism triggered by emotional disturbances works in the opposite way. When your child experiences increased stress and anxiety, it puts the sympathetic nervous system in overdrive. The body perceives this situation as a crisis and initiates the coping or supporting mechanism of hoarding resources to combat the crisis. Unfortunately, fat and sugar are the easiest energy resources for the body to start accumulating. This response develops into obesity or diabetes. These children often find sweet and greasy foods to be comforting while under stress or emotional crisis, further adding to the problem. The increased weight affects a child's quality of life due to lethargy, exhaustion, breathlessness, an excess load on weight-bearing joints, and social discrimination.

Ayurveda suggests that only a comprehensive approach of management can provide a sustainable outcome. That includes diet, lifestyle practices, activity, breathing techniques, and mind management techniques like counseling. Ayurvedic principles for managing obesity in children focus on a reduction of kapha coupled with streamlining agni. While approaches to weight loss that include drastic crash diets or excessive exercise may provide a sudden drop in body weight, this path will only lead to instant gratification; it will never provide a sustainable outcome and may affect the balanced growth and development of your child. Ayurveda recommends taking a moderate and consistent approach using as many tools as possible. The tools Dr. J finds most effective for supporting and managing obesity in children are:

1. Offer your children balanced and satisfying meals three times a day with varied ingredients like lentils, vegetables, whole grains, proteins, and spices, and reduce sweets, oils, and fatty items. This will help them feel satiated and engage the entire digestive system in a normal and gradual digestive process without a sudden surge of carbohydrates to the system. Regular mealtimes support the body's natural intelligence to align the digestive and metabolic systems with circadian rhythms to perform optimally and enhance the reutilization of fat in the body.

2. Create moderate and consistent daily activities and engage your children in outdoor games based on their interests. Simple and consistent activities every day will provide more sustainable results than excessive exercise two or three times a week.

3. Specific pranayama techniques or breathing practices with activating breaths like Kapalabhati or the Breath of Fire can be very helpful when performed regularly for a few minutes. Children should not engage in breathing practices immediately after meals. It is ideal to wait an hour after eating.

4. Children who have a tendency for emotional eating need to be supported to manage their stress and emotional issues through active interventions by parents that create opportunities to have positive conversations and facilitate practices like meditation and journaling.

5. There are many Ayurvedic natural herbs and formulations that can support obesity by enhancing digestion and metabolism and streamlining the metabolic and energy hormones, which can be

incorporated into a treatment protocol based on the guidance of an Ayurvedic physician.

A healthy diet, regular physical activity, and positive lifestyle practices can help children achieve and maintain a healthy weight starting at an early age that continues throughout their lives.

Diabetes

Diabetes comes under a group of diseases called prameha in Ayurvedic medicine. The literal translation of the word *prameha* is "passing large amounts of urine." There are twenty types of prameha: ten kapha-predominant, six related to pitta, and four associated with vata aggravation.

Excessive urination and turbidity (cloudiness) are the common features of all stages of prameha, considered a heterogeneous group of diseases with a common symptom of increased production of urine with sweetness and altered viscosity. The involvement of all the doshas along with diabetes's strong connection to vital organs like the pancreas (*kloma*) and urinary system (*vasti*) makes it a serious illness with a prolonged nature and various complications.

Both type 1 and type 2 diabetes can initiate at any age. Children are more prone to type 1. In this case, the pancreas doesn't produce sufficient insulin so that the body is unable to utilize sugars including glucose, causing an increase of sugar levels in the blood. Type 2 diabetes used to be considered strictly "adult onset" diabetes as children weren't as prone to it, but the drastic increase in childhood obesity has led to more children being diagnosed with type 2 diabetes these days. The most common reasons type 2 diabetes presents in children are being overweight, hereditary reasons, having a mother who had diabetes during pregnancy, or diseases that affect insulin production. Improper diet and lifestyle contribute to this condition.

According to Ayurvedic principles, the disease processes of diabetes and obesity have many similarities, and children with obesity are prone to diabetes and vice versa. The various reasons mentioned above cause weakened agni, which in turn affects the body's efficiency in processing food and absorbing nutrients into tissues, energy, and vitality. The unutilized food and nutrients accumulate in the body, causing further stagnation and weakness, and the sustained presence of increased sugar levels in the blood affects the consistency of the body fluids, causing increased drainage through the kidneys or excessive urination (polyuria) and excessive thirst (polydipsia). These fluid imbalances and metabolic irregularities then begin to affect vital organs leading to further diabetic complications including vision problems (diabetic retinopathy) and degeneration of nerves (diabetic neuropathy).

Ayurvedic management of prameha is not just about reducing blood sugar. Ayurveda's focus is to correct the root cause: enhancing agni, removing stagnation (*ama*), and correcting system irregularities. A carefully planned healing protocol with a balanced diet, regular activities, streamlined lifestyle practices, and traditional Ayurvedic herbs and formulations are all brought to bear.

Certain food ingredients and spices are considered very beneficial for managing diabetes. Bitter melon has been proven to have positive effects in controlling diabetes but, because of the palatability issue, requires preparing simple dishes for children rather than consuming the juice or soup of bitter melon directly. Ayurveda considers the combination of Indian gooseberry powder and turmeric powder the best home remedy (*agrya oushadha*) for prameha. A common practice is to drink half a cup of warm water with ½ teaspoon of Indian gooseberry powder and ¼ teaspoon of turmeric powder a day. Common spices like fenugreek seed, black cumin, Indian curry leaves, and turmeric powder are all suggested for children with diabetes. Daily physical activities, kapha-reducing breathing techniques, eating according to a set schedule, staying clear of simple carbohydrates, and avoiding daytime sleep as well as staying up too late are some specific guidelines for all individuals with diabetes.

There are many other disorders that can affect the digestive and metabolic systems. The Ayurvedic system of medicine focuses on correcting the body system regardless of symptoms or the name of a specific condition or disorder. You can understand the management principles of all possible disorders in a single system the same way. Since digestion and metabolism or agni are Ayurveda's main consideration for prevention as well as healing all diseases, learning about imbalances of the digestive and metabolic system can help you understand and create protocols for other system disorders as well.

15

RESPIRATORY DISORDERS

AYURVEDA IDENTIFIES THE respiratory system as *pranavaha srotas,* meaning "that which carries the vital breath that provides the subtle energies of prana and supports sustenance of life." Hence the saying: life starts with a breath and ends with a breath! Ayurvedic science assigns great importance to the management of respiratory disorders as these conditions not only cause distressing symptoms, such as struggling for breath, but also affect the growth and development of children as well as their resistance to other diseases and longevity.

Earaches

Being in their kapha cycle of life, children tend to have increased secretions of mucus and lots of congestion that leaves them susceptible to different types of earaches, known as *karnasoola* in Ayurveda. In addition to that, children's eustachian tubes—the passageway that connects the middle ear to the upper part of the throat—are narrower than an adult's, which can often lead to blockages and dysfunction. Have your children ever experienced severe earaches when taking off or landing during air travel? When the eustachian tubes become blocked with mucus, it causes difficulty regulating and equalizing the pressure inside the middle ear to the air pressure outside of the body, the primary reason children have pain when flying.

Middle ear infections (otitis media) are another common reason for earaches in children due to retention and accumulation of mucus in the middle ear—the space behind the eardrum—that often triggers inflammation and infections. Earaches due to otitis media usually last a few days and can be accompanied by a fever. This type of infection can sometimes lead to complications like a ruptured eardrum or discharge of pus from the ear, a condition Ayurveda refers to as *pootikarna* that expresses as purulent discharge with a foul smell due to pus formation. Other common causes of earaches are swimmer's ear (otitis externa), injury of the ear canal from a Q-tip or fingernail, accumulation of earwax blocking the ear canal, and a foreign body in the ear canal. While pain is an obvious indication of an ear infection or disorder, there are other common symptoms to watch for:

- Dull, sharp, or throbbing pain in the ear
- Discharge from the ear
- Itching in the ear
- Ringing or hissing sounds (tinnitus)
- Loss of hearing
- Feeling that the ear is blocked or trouble hearing

Ayurveda distinguishes different types of earaches based on doshic expressions. Vata-related ear disorders typically include severe pain associated with thin or no discharge, dry earwax, ringing in the ears (tinnitus), and loss of hearing. Pitta earaches express redness, swelling, burning, hypersensitivity, and yellow discharge with pus. Kapha types are characterized by swelling, itching, white or slimy discharge, and dull ache.

The Ayurvedic management of earaches includes avoiding known causes such as swimming and exposure to cold, supporting the ear channels to relieve blockages and congestion, healing existing inflammation and infection, and, finally, enhancing immune resistance to prevent tendencies toward congestion and avoid recurrence. Here are the most important tips for managing earaches in children:

1. Avoid washing your child's hair or wetting their head as soon as your child expresses initial symptoms of ear problems such as a feeling the ear is heavy or blocked. As Ayurveda considers the head to be the seat of kapha dosha, wetting the scalp can always cause an increased chance of congestion and heaviness. For children who experience repeated ear problems, it is recommended they minimize the frequency of head wetting in general.

2. Avoid cold food and beverages. Cold always aggravates kapha and vata; increased kapha causes congestion, whereas aggravated vata increases tendencies of pain.

3. If your child experiences earaches when flying, guide them to repeatedly swallow their spit or chew gum during takeoff and landing as the action of swallowing can help open the eustachian tube and avoid pressure changes inside the middle ear. Another helpful exercise is to ask your child to inhale deeply and fill the mouth with air like a balloon for a few seconds without exhaling.

4. Gargle with warm salt water two or three times a day. The practice of gargling with warm water with a high concentration of salt can relieve the swelling and congestion in the ears through osmosis and quickly reduce earaches.

5. Avoid late nights as this causes aggravation of vata and any pain your child may be experiencing. Daytime sleep is also discouraged as it can cause kapha aggravation and more congestion.

6. Avoid cleaning your child's ears with Q-tips when they have an earache as the ear is very sensitive and the intensity of pain can increase with pressure. It is always advisable to consult with an expert to manage such issues.

7. There are many specific Ayurvedic herbs and formulations that can be taken internally and also used in combination with external therapies and local applications. An Ayurvedic physician can personalize a treatment protocol for your child.

Tonsillitis

Tonsillitis is very common in children and known as *tundikeri* in Ayurveda, a condition characterized by inflammation of the tonsils, the lumps of lymphoid tissues on both sides of the back of the throat. Ayurveda recognizes tonsillitis as an indication the immune system is fighting against a possible infection that may affect the body. In the active stage of tonsillitis, if you look inside your child's mouth, the red, swollen tonsils will be visible in the throat. Tonsillitis causes severe pain that can even make it difficult for your child to swallow their own spit. Many children get recurrent tonsillitis that can develop into other issues including severe fever, losing their voice, difficulty swallowing, and earache if left untreated.

The tonsils play a key role in our health fighting off germs that can enter the body through the nose and mouth and lead to infection. They are considered part of the lymphatic system and function as a component of the body's active immune defense mechanisms that pool defense cells when there is a high probability of invading pathogenic organisms. This fight against invading viruses or pathogenic bacteria causes swelling and inflammation. Tonsillitis can produce white or yellow discharge and can sometimes be accompanied by enlarged adenoids. ENTs used to commonly recommend that children with recurrent tonsillitis have surgery to remove the tonsils (tonsillectomy), but that is becoming less frequent these days as there is no evidence that having a tonsillectomy reduces the chance of infections in children. In fact, removing the tonsils is like removing the front door of your house, allowing anybody and anything to enter without warning or barrier.

Ayurveda considers your child's mild fevers and occasional sore throat an indication their immune defenses are becoming more active. Such exposures to possible threats from pathogens gradually make the body's resistance to infections stronger. As your child's immune system develops resistance, you can manage and prevent mild illnesses at home with some basic regimens and home remedies. Ayurveda explains that exposures to cold wind, intake of cold food or beverages, cold showers, or even cold and moist weather can trigger tonsillitis. The most common symptoms are:

- Swelling inside the throat with redness and pain
- Pain while swallowing
- Fever and chills
- Loss of voice and bad breath
- Sore throat

The management of tundikeri in Ayurveda not only provides symptomatic relief but also treats the current condition and prevents the chances of recurrence. Here are the most common tips and home remedies to prevent and manage tonsillitis:

1. Minimize wetting the head, especially for children who have a tendency to get tonsillitis. Cold water on the head, the seat of kapha, can cause increased congestion and tonsil inflammation.
2. Avoid eating cold food and drinking cold beverages as cold aggravates both kapha and vata.
3. Sipping lukewarm water with fresh squeezed lemon juice, raw honey, and a pinch of salt throughout the day is found to be supportive to reduce inflammation and keep symptoms from progressing.
4. Gargling with warm water that has a slightly higher concentration of salt multiple times a day can reduce swelling and relieve difficulty swallowing instantaneously.
5. Regular intake of warm cow's milk with ¼ teaspoon turmeric powder and a touch of black pepper is Dr. J's favorite home remedy to support children who tend to get recurrent tonsillitis.
6. Gargling with water boiled with leaves of holy basil with salt and turmeric during the active stage of tonsillitis is sometimes found to be helpful.
7. There are specific Ayurvedic herbs like lilac tasselflower (*Emilia sonchifolia*) and traditional formulations that can be taken to manage tonsillitis and related issues based on the advice of an Ayurvedic physician. Rejuvenators (rasayana) like Chyawanprash are commonly used by parents at home to help strengthen their child's resistance against recurrent inflammations.

Flu

Flu, or influenza, is a contagious viral infection that affects the nose, throat, and lungs and spreads through droplets when people with flu cough, talk, or sneeze. While flu is primarily a respiratory infection, it can lead to other complications and sometimes be fatal. Ayurveda classifies flu in the category of *kapha-vata jwara*, fever or inflammation caused by aggravation of kapha and vata. When flu isn't managed well in the initial stages, it can affect the upper respiratory tract and cause sinusitis or move to the lower respiratory tract (lungs), causing cough and chest congestion. Flu can progress into bacterial infections like pneumonia, sinus infections, and ear infections. Ayurveda identifies conditions like flu as an indication of reduced vitality and immune resistance (*bala*) in children. This is the reason children don't all develop flu-like symptoms when one or two individuals in a classroom invariably present with a runny nose, sneezing, coughing, and are likely spreading droplets to everyone. Flu typically starts with a sudden onset of the following symptoms:

- Sore throat
- Nasal congestion and runny nose
- Aches and pains in the body with headaches
- Fever with chills
- Heaviness of head with extreme tiredness
- Children can also develop vomiting and diarrhea
- Cough and chest congestion

The Ayurvedic management of flu includes taking precautions to avoid close contact with people who are sick with flu, carefully managing the initial onset with care to minimize the development of symptoms and progression, and supporting children to enhance immune resistance to prevent such infections. The most effective Ayurvedic tips for preventing and managing flu are to reduce further imbalances of vata and kapha, the doshas primarily involved in this condition. Here are some ways you can modify your child's lifestyle to support recovery:

1. Avoid cold food and beverages.
2. Minimize exposure to cold, and make sure your child wears layers in cold weather and seasons to protect them from prolonged exposure.
3. Avoid cold showers.
4. Make sure you towel-dry your child's scalp after hair washing as a wet scalp can trigger sneezing, runny nose, and congestion.
5. Avoid late nights.

When you see initial symptoms of flu in your child like sore throat, sneezing, or congestion, the following Ayurvedic tips can be helpful:

1. Allow your child to rest completely.
2. Offer only easily digestible, warm cooked food like soups.
3. Avoid hair washing for a few days.
4. Boil three or four leaves of holy basil in a cup of water for five minutes, adding a teaspoon of honey once it cools down to lukewarm, and have your child sip throughout the day.
5. Prepare a mixture of ¼ teaspoon turmeric powder with one teaspoon of honey and a touch of black pepper powder. Give this to your child in three or four divided doses in one day.
6. Have them sip warm ginger tea made with two or three slices of fresh ginger in a cup of water to relieve congestion and clear the respiratory channels.
7. Gargle with warm salt water to reduce swelling and congestion.

Ayurveda's main focus is to support children to avoid recurrent colds and flu. There are many home remedies and Ayurvedic herbs and formulations you can use to support your children's immune health:

1. The regular intake of herbs like turmeric and ashwagandha in hot milk (golden milk) has been found to be supportive to enhance immune strength.
2. Traditional formulations like Indukantham Ghritam, Amalaki Rasayana, and Chyawanprash have been used for centuries to enhance immune resistance in children.

Asthma

Asthma is a serious, chronic respiratory disease that can severely affect the health of growing children. Bronchial asthma is known as *tamaka shwasa* in Ayurveda and leads to abnormal breathing patterns, difficulty breathing, chest tightness, wheezing, and coughing. Children who have a tendency toward asthma can easily develop inflammation of the lungs and airways when they are exposed to causative factors or when they have conditions like cold or flu. Since asthma affects the airways and oxygen levels, it impacts a child's overall activity, growth, and quality of life. Ayurveda identifies asthma as a condition developed due to aggravations of vata and kapha doshas, as well as pitta at certain stages. There are many known causes for asthma, and it varies for every child. The most common triggers are:

- Allergic asthma is one of the most common types of asthma in children when the respiratory system reacts to different irritants and exposures. When a child inhales an allergen, their immune system perceives a crisis, and the body's response is to constrict the respiratory airways (bronchioles), causing restricted airflow to the lungs. This presents as breathlessness and difficulty getting the required oxygen to the system. As a consequence, there can be acute inflammation of the respiratory tract that leads to increased secretion of mucus and further closure of the breath channels. Dust mites, pollen, molds, cockroaches, and pet dander are some of the most common respiratory allergens that affect children.

- Air pollution or irritants in the air is another common reason for childhood asthma. Wood fires, charcoal grills, cigarette smoke, fumes from vaping, air pollution such as smog, strong chemicals, dust, and fumes are known to aggravate inflamed and sensitive respiratory channels. A child doesn't necessarily need to be allergic to these exposures to become symptomatic, but the intensity and sharpness of these items creates irritation of the mucosal lining of the respiratory system.

- Asthma can also develop as a symptom of other underlying disorders and diseases in children that create inflammation, constriction, and inflammation of the airways such as: obstructive sleep apnea, acid reflux (GERD), obesity, chronic obstructive pulmonary disease (COPD), nasal polyps, pneumonia, flu, sinusitis, and rhinitis.
- Exercise-induced asthma is another condition that can develop in children, which may only appear after prolonged and sustained exercise. Dr. J has seen many cases where children exposed to extreme training as a part of a competitive sports program experienced symptoms of bronchoconstriction (EIB), especially in cold weather.
- Certain strong emotions in children can trigger asthma-like symptoms. These strong emotions can cause changes to breathing patterns and bring on wheezing even when a child doesn't have a history of asthma. Fear, anger, laughter, crying, feeling insecure, excitement, and yelling are some of the emotional triggers that may cause symptoms of asthma.
- Weather can also trigger asthma in certain children. Sudden changes in weather, dry wind, cold air, cloudy conditions, and thunderstorms are known to cause asthma symptoms in some children. Seasonal asthma is mainly due to specific allergens like pollen that get released into the atmosphere.
- Chemical medications such as certain anti-inflammatory drugs and beta-blockers can trigger symptoms of asthma in some children.

The signs and symptoms of childhood asthma can vary from child to child, and sometimes change from one episode to the next. The most common signs and symptoms are:

- Fast and difficult breathing
- Pain and tightness in chest
- Whistling sound while breathing in or out (wheezing)
- Persistent cough that doesn't go away

- Episodes of continuous coughing that occur often, especially at night, during exercise or physical activity, from exposure to cold air, or from crying or laughing
- Reduced energy during play, and needing to take breaks during physical activities to catch their breath
- Avoidance or lack of desire to participate in sports or physical activities
- Difficulty in lying flat and sleeping due to cough or breathing difficulties

The vata-predominant stage of asthma expresses as dry cough, breathing difficulty due to airway constriction without phlegm, wheezing, pain in the chest, and difficulty talking and sleeping. In the kapha stage there will be increased white, thick mucus as well as chest heaviness with congestion. A pitta association is comparatively rare, but yellowish or greenish mucus and sometimes phlegm stained with blood are all indications.

Ayurvedic management of childhood asthma varies according to the type of asthma as well as which dosha is predominant at that time. The overall approach of management is multipronged with dietary and lifestyle guidance, herbs and formulations to stabilize the condition, and administration of rejuvenators specific to supporting the respiratory system as well as enhancing immune resistance. Ayurvedic guidance for parents to support children with asthma is as follows:

1. The first step of managing allergic asthma is to avoid or limit exposure to the allergens. It will be challenging to avoid the allergens completely when it comes to pollen or air pollutants. Keeping the windows closed, using filtering masks when exposed to the external environment, and employing quality air purifiers are some of the practical options to minimize the exposures.
2. Avoid eating cold food, drinking cold beverages, and taking cold showers as cold aggravates both kapha and vata.
3. Sipping warm water with heating spices like ginger throughout the day is found to be supportive as warmth always dilates and cold always constricts.

4. Regular intake of warm cow's milk with ¼ teaspoon turmeric powder and a touch of black pepper is known to help reduce tendencies of respiratory allergies in children.

5. Sipping water boiled with leaves of holy basil with turmeric powder and raw honey is found to be helpful. Ayurveda suggests never heating honey and only adding it to tea that is lukewarm. Incorporating ingredients like garlic, turmeric, ginger, and black pepper when preparing meals can help reduce vata and kapha and lower tendencies of asthma.

6. Restrict cold and hard to digest foods as well as ingredients such as yogurt, oil, fried items, black lentils, and fish as these can aggravate vata and kapha, causing more constriction and congestion.

7. There are specific Ayurvedic herbs like long pepper (*pippali*), licorice root (yashtimadhu), ashwagandha, and traditional formulations, which can be taken based on the advice from an Ayurvedic doctor to manage childhood asthma and associated problems. Rejuvenators (rasayana) like Chyawanprash have specific indications to support respiratory issues and help the body's resistance against immune sensitivities and inflammation.

8. Ayurveda recommends external applications of heat such as steam and warm towels and herbal oils like Karpuradi Thailam to help relieve chest tightness during an active asthma attack.

As we have discussed, children are especially prone to respiratory issues as they are in the kapha period of life, and this is the primary reason Ayurveda suggests avoiding exposures to cold in any form whether as a cold shower or drinking cold water. Since the respiratory system provides the vital life force energy of prana and facilitates metabolism and sustained energy, any issues that hinder the respiratory system affect children in a much deeper way than adults. It is essential that parents take necessary precautions to support their children's health and avoid recurrent respiratory issues as the most common conditions in childhood.

16

AYURVEDIC HOME REMEDIES

"LET THY FOOD be thy medicine, and medicine be thy food" is often ascribed to the Greek physician Hippocrates; however, the wisdom of Ayurvedic healing has considered food a powerful medicine since the ancient Indian Vedic period (1500–500 BCE). Ayurveda's approach to health and longevity includes various home remedies and recipes using food, herbs, spices, medicinal plants, and formulated oils along with nutritional healing principles to support the body to resist disease, recover from disorders, and prevent recurring symptoms and illnesses.

If you've ever wished for a little help from Mother Nature to treat your children's everyday common complaints, traditional Ayurvedic home remedies can offer you and your family plenty of natural relief. In fact, you can find most of the ingredients you need to follow simple, common Ayurvedic recipes right in your kitchen cabinets and backyard or window-sill garden! When you take action in the early stages of any health issue, you can help avoid further progression of ailments and disorders and promote healing at initial stages, relieve symptoms, and restore balance to the mind-body system.

Many parents today prefer gentler, holistic remedies for an integrated model of care in relationship with modern medicine whenever possible.

Ayurveda provides a series of natural healing techniques and therapies you can easily implement at home that offer convenience, a low risk of side effects, and cost-effective solutions to keep your children's minds and bodies healthy. From sleep tonics to stomachaches, you will find many useful recipes in the following sections to support alleviating common everyday ailments in combination with the lifestyle routines and Ayurvedic regimens you have discovered throughout this book.

Introducing New Flavors

Before you jump into experimenting with different recipes, Dr. J shares some practical advice on the best ways to introduce new flavors and ingredients to your children. This will help you steer clear of resistance so you can make the most of these natural health remedies!

Throughout his Ayurvedic practice, Dr. J has found it is often much easier to work with children than adults because of their simple, open-minded nature. They do not have the same preconceived ideas that we do as adults and are generally more acceptant and even curious about new practices and routines presented to them. What matters most is not what you introduce, but how you introduce something new, whether it is an herb, a formulation, or a new recipe. When you follow principles that gradually acquaint your children with unfamiliar tastes, they will tolerate different remedies without difficulty and make it easier for you to regularly introduce effective, natural remedies at home.

First, always start with the minimal quantity when introducing a new taste and gradually build up to the recommended amount. If a recipe calls for 1/2 teaspoon as the full dosage, for example, start with a few drops mixed in with something you know your child enjoys. As they slowly get used to the flavor, you can gradually increase to the usual measurement over a few days. When you give a child an initial full dose of an unfamiliar taste, as you probably know from your own experience, there is a high likelihood an aversion will set in that will be challenging at best to overcome.

The second rule of thumb is to sweeten the deal—combining new tastes, especially when bitter or astringent with more palatable accompaniments like honey or maple syrup make it easy for kids to try something new. Once they get used to the flavors and tastes of new herbs and spices, treating ailments at home with simple ingredients will become second nature for everyone.

Colds and Congestion

TULSI GINGER TEA WITH HONEY

Prep time: 10–15 minutes

INGREDIENTS

1 cup water

¼ teaspoon grated fresh or dried ginger

¼ teaspoon tulsi (holy basil) leaf powder (or 2 fresh leaves if available)

¼ teaspoon black pepper powder

1 teaspoon (or as needed) raw honey or palm jaggery

Boil the water with the grated or powdered ginger, tulsi, and black pepper powder for 5 minutes. Remove from the stove, allow to cool down to lukewarm, add raw honey or palm jaggery, and offer in 2–4 divided doses once every 3–4 hours.

TURMERIC GINGER CUMIN TEA

Prep time: 10–15 minutes

INGREDIENTS

1 cup water

¼ teaspoon grated fresh or dried ginger

¼ teaspoon cumin seed

¼ teaspoon turmeric powder

1 teaspoon (or as needed) raw honey

Boil the water with the grated or powdered ginger, cumin seed, and turmeric powder for 5 minutes. Remove from the stove, allow to cool down to lukewarm, add raw honey, and offer in 2–4 divided doses once every 2–3 hours.

Dry Cough with Sore Throat

PEARL ONION, LEMON, AND HONEY
Prep time: 10 minutes
INGREDIENTS
1 pink pearl onion
½ fresh lemon or lime
1 tablespoon raw honey

Chop the pearl onion into small slices and place in a small bowl. Squeeze half a lemon or lime into the chopped pearl onion. Add the raw honey and mix it very well. Give ¼ teaspoon of this mixture every hour.

Respiratory Allergies and Immunity Booster

GOLDEN MILK WITH SAFFRON
Prep time: 10–15 minutes
INGREDIENTS
1 cup organic whole milk
¼ teaspoon turmeric powder
Palm jaggery or unrefined cane sugar, to taste (optional)
4–6 threads saffron (optional)

Boil the milk with the turmeric and palm jaggery or unrefined cane sugar. Add the saffron when you remove the milk from the heat. Offer to your child at bedtime.

Drinking warm milk at bedtime is known to enhance the quality of sleep. Children are more prone to kapha dosha aggravations, and the warmth of turmeric and saffron helps to cut the kapha-increasing nature of the milk. Turmeric is also traditionally known to enhance immune resistance against allergies.

Disturbed Sleep

MILK WITH NUTMEG

Prep time: 10 minutes

INGREDIENTS

1 cup organic whole milk

1 small pinch nutmeg powder

1 teaspoon (or as needed) unrefined cane sugar

Bring the milk to a boil with a pinch of nutmeg powder. Add the unrefined cane sugar as needed. Drink while still warm, ideally at bedtime.

Constipation

MILK WITH CANE JAGGERY

Prep Time: 10 minutes

INGREDIENTS

1 cup organic whole milk

1 teaspoon cane jaggery

Boil the milk and mix in the jaggery. Drink at bedtime. It usually helps with easy elimination the next day.

Dehydration

MINT LEMONADE WITH SWEET AND SALT

Prep time: 5 minutes

INGREDIENTS

1 cup water

2 tablespoons unrefined cane sugar

¼ teaspoon sea salt

3 mint leaves, chopped

½ lemon or lime

Mix 2 tablespoons of sugar into room temperature water, then add ¼ teaspoon salt and 3 chopped mint leaves. Squeeze half of a lemon into the glass, mix well, and serve fresh. You can adjust the sweet and salt based on your child's palate. This is good to serve to kids while playing intense sports or when they come back after their workouts or outdoor games.

COCONUT WATER WITH CARDAMOM
Prep time: 5 minutes
INGREDIENTS
1 cup coconut water
1 teaspoon unrefined cane sugar
1 pinch (about 1 gram) cardamom powder

Dissolve the unrefined cane sugar in the coconut water, then add 1 pinch of cardamom powder to it. Mix well and serve fresh.

Diarrhea and Nausea

ARROWROOT SOUP
Prep time: 15 minutes
INGREDIENTS
1 tablespoon arrowroot powder
1 cup water
1 pinch cumin powder
Himalayan pink salt to taste

Boil the arrowroot in the water with cumin powder over medium heat until it becomes a thick liquid consistency. Serve warm after adding salt to taste.

LEMON, GINGER, AND HONEY

Prep time: 10 minutes

INGREDIENTS

½ lemon or lime

1 cup filtered water or boiled and cooled water

½ teaspoon fresh ginger juice

¼ teaspoon sea salt

Squeeze the lemon or lime into the water. Add the ginger juice with the salt, and stir well. Give in divided doses once every 2 hours. Once the appetite returns to normal, serve rice soup with a pinch of salt for hydration and strength.

RICE SOUP

Prep time: 20 minutes

INGREDIENTS

1 tablespoon basmati rice

1½–2 cups water

A pinch of salt, ginger, or cumin to taste

Boil 1 tablespoon of rice with 1½–2 cups of water until the rice is soft and well-cooked. Serve warm with a pinch of salt to taste and additional spices, such as a pinch of ginger or cumin powder, as desired.

POMEGRANATE ORANGE PEEL TEA

Prep time: 15 minutes

INGREDIENTS

1 teaspoon chopped pomegranate peel

½ teaspoon chopped orange or lemon peel

2 cups filtered water or boiled and cooled water

Boil the peels of the pomegranate and orange or lemon in the water for 3–5 minutes. Allow tea to cool down to lukewarm and then give 1 tablespoon every hour.

Indigestion

GINGER TEA WITH JAGGERY

Prep time: 10 minutes

INGREDIENTS

1 cup water

¼ teaspoon grated fresh or dried ginger

1 teaspoon (or as needed for taste) cane jaggery

Boil the water with the grated or powdered ginger for 5 minutes. Remove from the stove, allow to cool down to lukewarm, and add the cane jaggery. Give it in 2–4 divided doses in a day.

POMEGRANATE JUICE WITH ROASTED CUMIN SEED

Prep time: 10 minutes

INGREDIENTS

1 tablespoon pomegranate juice

1 pinch (about 1 gram) dry roasted cumin seed powder

½ teaspoon raw honey

Take the pomegranate juice, and mix in a pinch of dry roasted cumin powder and raw honey. Give it before a meal.

Abdominal Pain/Colic

CAROM SEED WATER

Prep time: 10 minutes

INGREDIENTS

1 cup water

¼ teaspoon carom seed powder

Boil the water and remove from the stove after it boils for 2 minutes. Allow it to cool down to lukewarm, then add the carom seed powder. Give in 3–4 divided doses in a day.

Ayurvedic Mouthwash

POMEGRANATE PEEL CARDAMOM MOUTH RINSE
Prep time: 15 minutes
INGREDIENTS
1 teaspoon chopped pomegranate peel
1 cup filtered water
1 pinch (about 1 gram) cardamom powder

Boil the pomegranate peels in the water for 3–5 minutes, and then allow to cool down to lukewarm. Add a pinch of cardamom powder and use for rinsing the mouth 2–3 times a day.

Bath Scrub

MUNG BEAN AND LICORICE PASTE
INGREDIENTS
1 tablespoon mung bean powder
1 teaspoon licorice powder
Water or organic whole milk, as needed

This common Ayurvedic scrub for children removes dirt and excess oil, keeps skin healthy, and prevents dryness from harsh soaps and body products. Combine the mung bean powder with the licorice powder and mix into a fine paste with a little water or milk. Apply this paste all over the body, massaging gently into skin, then wash off for glowing clean skin.

Traditional Ayurvedic Oils for Children

Ayurvedic herbal oils are an important part of the daily routine for all constitution types and have various healing benefits. Consult the following index of natural oil formulations to promote whole-body healing and rejuvenation, relieve physical discomfort, and balance the doshas.

Oil	Mode of Application	Effect on Dosha	Traditional Uses
Balahatadi Keram	Head massage	V↓P↓	Headaches, migraines
Balaswagandhadi Thailam	Whole body massage	V↓P↓	Tissue building, nourishing, and strengthening
Bala Thailam	Whole body massage	V↓	General nourishment and balance
Chandanadi Thailam	Body and scalp massage	P↓	Burning sensations in the body and scalp
Chandanadi Thailam	Head massage	P↓V↓	Insomnia, anxiety
Chemparathyadi Keram	Body and scalp massage	P↓V↓	Skin diseases, itchy scalp
Dharani	Whole body massage	K↓V↓	Warming and cleansing
Dinesa Keram	Local application	V↓P↓	Good for sensitive skin, healing wounds, and skin conditions
Durvadi Keram	Local application	V↓P↓	Eczema
Eladi Keram	Body and scalp massage	V↓K↓	Itchy skin conditions, dark circles, and skin blemishes
Karpuradi Thailam	Local application	V↓	Soothes muscles spasms and helps ease growing pains
Kayyunyadi Keram	Scalp massage	V↓P↓K↓	Supports hair growth and relieves dandruff
Kesini	Scalp massage	V↓P↓	Complete scalp and hair care, relieves dandruff, and eases alopecia

Oil	Mode of Application	Effect on Dosha	Traditional Uses
Ksheerabala Thailam	Whole body massage	V↓P↓	Calms the nerves; nourishing and soothing
Lakshadi Thailam	Whole body massage	V↓P↓	Massage oil for kids, bone healing, and strengthening
Mahachandanadi Thailam	Scalp massage	P↓	Most cooling oil; relieves stress and supports anxiety
Mahamasha Thailam	Whole body massage	V↓	Nourishes muscles and nerves
Mahanarayana Thailam	Whole body massage	V↓	Strengthening and nourishing
Murivenna	Local application	V↓P↓	Help heal tissue injuries, fungal infections
Nalpamaradi	Local application	K↓P↓	Skin conditions like eczema
Neelibringadi Keram	Head massage	P↓	Total hair care
Pavan	Whole body massage	V↓	Calms the mind and strengthens the body
Pinda Thailam	Whole body massage	V↓ P↓	Most moistening oil; helps cracked feet and dry skin
Santhwanam	Whole body massage	V↓P↓K↓	Improves blood circulation, skin quality, and vitality
Tejas	Whole body massage	P↓	Cools burning sensations and dry skin
Triphaladi	Head massage	V↓P↓K↓	Good for hair, skin, and eye health
Winsoria	Local application	V↓	Soothes itchy flaky skin, psoriasis, eczema, and dandruff

CONCLUSION

WE ARE MOST grateful to have shared in your wellness journey, and it is our hope that we have inspired you along the way to discover the many simple ways you can live in accordance with Ayurvedic principles. The intention of this book was to introduce the basic principles of Ayurveda into your life and show you the many simple ways you can customize your family's wellness routines. Our hope is to set you on a path where you feel empowered to embrace Ayurveda as a way of life, creating and maintaining health and balance so you and your children can attain the highest quality of life possible and reach your greatest potential. Simply put, the goal of Ayurveda is to live a long, healthy, harmonious, happy, and peaceful life.

We are passionate about supporting communities individually and collectively at Kerala Ayurveda and remain a continued resource for enhancing your family's wellness. Along with consultations to personalize Ayurvedic regimens for children and adults under the guidance of an experienced Ayurvedic practitioner, you will find many supports at Kerala including a wide range of Ayurvedic products and traditional formulations you have discovered in this book, family and youth wellness courses, and many other programs that invite you to deepen your knowledge of Ayurveda.

NOTES

CHAPTER 6. BREATH

1. "Yoga and Breathing Exercises Aid Children with ADHD to Focus," Ural Federal University, May 16, 2021, https://neurosciencenews.com/focus -yoga-adhd-18435.

CHAPTER 8. SLEEP

1. Michael Breus, "The Sleep Benefits of Ayurvedic Medicine," *Psychology Today*, August 2020, https://www.psychologytoday.com/us/blog/sleep -newzzz/202008/the-sleep-benefits-ayurvedic-medicine.
2. G. M. Nixon, J. M. Thompson, D. Y. Han, D. M. Becroft, P. M. Clark, E. Robinson, K. E. Waldie, C. J. Wild, P. N. Black, E. A. Mitchell, "Falling Asleep: The Determinants of Sleep Latency," *Archives of Disease in Childhood* 94, no. 9 (September 2009): 686–89, https://doi.org/10.1136/adc.2009.157453.

CHAPTER 11. YOGA, MEDITATION, AND MANTRAS FOR KIDS

1. "Research on Mindfulness," Mindful Schools (website), accessed August 2021, https://www.mindfulschools.org/about-mindfulness/research-on -mindfulness/#reference-22.
2. "Introduce Yoga to Your Children for Health, Happiness, and Better Concentration," National Commission for Protection of Child Rights (New Delhi, India), 2–3, https://ncpcr.gov.in/showfile.php?lang=1&level =1&&sublinkid=1566&lid=1639.
3. "Just Breathe: The Importance of Meditation Breaks for Kids," Healthy Children (website), last updated April 19, 2017, https://www.healthychildren .org/English/healthy-living/emotional-wellness/Pages/Just-Breathe-The -Importance-of-Meditation-Breaks-for-Kids.aspx.
4. Crystal Raypole, "Have Trouble Meditating? Try Mantra Meditation," Healthline, August 18, 2020, https://www.healthline.com/health/mantra -meditation#takeaway.

5. C. R. Karnick, "Effect of Mantras on Human Beings and Plants," *Ancient Science of Life* 2, no. 3 (January–March 1983): 141–47, https://www.ncbi .nlm.nih.gov/pmc/articles/PMC3336746/.

CHAPTER 13. MIND-RELATED DISORDERS

1. "What Is Epigenetics?" Centers for Disease Control and Prevention, last updated August 3, 2020, https://www.cdc.gov/genomics/disease/epigenetics .htm.

CHAPTER 14. DIGESTIVE AND METABOLIC DISORDERS

1. Cheryl D. Fryar, Margaret D. Carroll, and Cynthia L. Ogden, "Prevalence of Overweight, Obesity, and Severe Obesity Among Children and Adolescents Aged 2–19 Years," Centers for Disease Control and Prevention, September 5, 2018, https://www.cdc.gov/nchs/data/hestat/obesity_child_15_16/obesity _child_15_16.htm.

INDEX

Tridosh pacifying, 109
for your child based on their dosha,
108–9
Breath of Fire (Kapalabhati), 108, 206
bronchial asthma *(tamaka shwasa)*, 217
bulimia, 202
bumblebee breath (Bhramari), 108, 109
bunny breath exercise, 109
Butterfly Pose, 157

calming breathwork, 102, 106–7, 108
calorie counting, 80–81
Camel Pose, 157
cane jaggery
food incompatibilities, 78
Ginger Tea with Jaggery, 228
Milk with Cane Jaggery, 225
cardamom
Coconut Water with Cardamom, 226
increasing *agni* with, 200
for nausea, vomiting, and diarrhea, 203
Pomegranate Peel Cardamom Mouth
Rinse, 229
for smoothies, 96
Carom Seed Water, 228
castor oil, 201
Cat Pose, 157, 158
CCF Tea, 90
cerebral palsy, 184
Chair Pose, 157, 158
chakras, 152, 169
Chandanadi Thailam oil, 230
Chandra Bhedana, 110
chanting mantras, 165–69
Chemparathyadi Keram oil, 230
child(ren) and childhood
balance of body, mind, and spirit in, 11
belly breathing with, 101–3
cell and tissue building/degeneration
during, 21–22
influence of kapha during, 45
kapha dosha and, 54–55
Kaumarabhritya and, 17–8
managing temptations and unhealthy
choices of, 178–79
mind-body-spirit connection in, 12–13,
25–26, 278
mind-body system in early, 18
mind of, 26–27, 115
monitoring digestion of, 82
parents' awareness of characteristics and
traits of, 29–30

perception in, 115–6
physiology and, 14–15
water intake, 85–86
See also kapha child(ren); pitta
child(ren); vata child(ren)
Child's Pose, 157
Chinmaya Mudra, 151
Chin Mudra, 151
choices, making unhealthy, 177–78
Chyawanprash, 214, 216, 220
circadian rhythms, 126, 129, 141, 142, 179
clove oil, 149
Cobra Pose, 157
coconut, 190
coconut oil, 128, 147, 148
coconut water, 139, 226
cognitive delays, 193
cold/cool food and beverages, 39, 40, 77
ADHD and, 189
allergies and, 60
asthma and, 219
colds/congestion and, 58
digestion and, 77
doshas and, 40
earaches and, 212
impact on health, 93–94, 96, 201
tonsillitis and, 214
colds and congestion, 45, 54, 58–59, 216,
219, 223
cold showers, 213, 216, 219
cold weather, 43, 45, 149, 213, 216, 218
colic/colicky abdominal pain, 185, 200, 201,
228
compassion, link between mindfulness and,
103
complementary and alternative medicine
(CAM), 20–21
computers, 118–19
conception, 16, 30, 193
congenital disease and factors, 175, 195
constipation, 108, 115, 136, 225
constitution. See *prakriti*
contraindications, 108, 109, 138, 145, 159–60
cooling breathwork, 107, 108
coriander/coriander seeds
in CCF Tea, 90
in Coriander Seed Tea, 91
supporting digestion, 75
for urinary complications, 70
co-sleeping, 131–32
Cow Pose, 157, 158
cumin/cumin seeds

peppermint, herbal tea blend using, 93
perception, 113–20
    in children, 115–16
    digital age and, 118–19
    disease and imbalanced, 177
    five senses and, 113, 115, 117–18
    function of, 68–69
    mindfulness and, 103
    restoring the senses and, 119
    trigunas and, 114–15
phakka (developmental delays), 193–94
physical activity. *See* exercise
physical (structural) aspect of existence, 2,
    21–23
physical body
    cell and tissue building/degeneration,
        21–22
    the five elements and, 40–41
    functional energies and, 22–23, 31
    trigunas expressed in, 114
    See also mind-body system
pichu, 183–84, 190, 192
Pinda Thailam oil, 231
pippali (long pepper), 220
pitta child(ren)
    breathing technique for, 107, 108
    characteristics of, 32, 35
    diet and, 73
    exercise and, 135, 137
    fluid intake, 95
    imbalance in, 158
    meditation for, 165
    sleep and, 128
    yoga for, 159
pitta dosha
    ADHD and, 189
    aggravating factors, 35
    characteristics of a balanced, 41
    cycle of life and, 45
    daily time cycles and, 44
    deficiency of, 24
    disorder tendencies with, 35
    early adulthood and, 45
    Fire element and, 41
    function of, 24
    principles of management with, 36
    seasonal influences, 43
    yoga and, 156
    See also doshas
pitta-kapha, 51, 52
pitta season, 137–38
pitta time of day/night, 126, 135, 143

plant-based diet, 83
pollens, 56, 59, 218
polydipsia, 208
polyuria, 208
pomegranate/pomegranate peel, 190, 203
    Pomegranate Juice with Roasted Cumin
        Seed, 228
    Pomegranate Orange Peel Tea, 227
    Pomegranate Peel Cardamom Mouth
        Rinse, 229
potential, at conception, 16
prakriti
    daily routines and, 142–44
    diet and, 72–73
    doshas and, 31–32
    explained, 30–31
    importance of understanding your
        child's, 31
    quiz for identifying your child's, 46–51
    See also doshas
prameha, 184, 207, 208
prana (life energy), 68, 101, 169
prana mantras, 169
pranayama, 153
    belly breathing, 101–3
    for nightmare and night terrors, 197
    for obesity, 206
    overview, 100–101
    See also breath and breathwork
pratyahara (withdrawal of senses), 153
prayer(s), 132, 164, 165, 166
preconception care, 190–91, 193
preschool age
    meditation for, 164
    yoga for, 162
principle of *chikitsa*, 180–82
principle of like increases like, 39–40, 42, 43
principle of *nidana*, 175–76
principle of opposites create balance, 39–40
principle of the six tastes, 73–74
probiotic supplements, 83–84
pruritus, 148
psoriasis, 62–63, 183
Psychology Today, 127
pungent (taste), 73, 74, 76

radishes, foods that are incompatible with,
    78
rajas, 114, 154, 164
Rasayana, 190
rasayanas (rejuvenating protocol), 61, 139,
    191, 214

focus on symptomatic relief of disease, 180–81
on mental health issues in children, 187
parents using complementary and alternative medicine with, 20–21
wheezing, 56, 57, 218, 219
whole-body oil massage
    for autism spectrum disorder, 192
    recommended oils and traditional uses for, 230, 231
    shashtika lepa, 182–83
    for sleep in vata children, 128
    for vata children, 128
    See also *abhyanga* (whole-body oil massage)
whole child, 3, 11, 13, 20–22
whole grains, 75, 206
wild Indian yam, 70
Wind Releasing Pose, 157
Winsoria oil, 231
winter melon, 69, 190
wintertime, 39, 43, 45, 55, 58, 137

yama, 153, 161
yashtimadhu (licorice root), 139, 195, 220

yoga
    for anxiety, 194–5, 195
    Ayurveda and, 153
    benefits of, 153, 154–55
    for children three to ten years old, 160–61
    developmental considerations for, 162
    doshas and, 136, 137, 153–54, 155–56, 158–59
    eight limbs of, 153–54
    guidelines for, 159–62
    introduced in the classroom, 152
    as natural-born ability in children, 151
    poses and postures for children, 155, 156, 157–58
    sample sequence for younger children, 157–58
    sleep and, 131
    for teens, 157, 158, 161
    tips for parents, 156–57
Yoga Nidra, 163–64, 195
yogurt, 62, 78, 220

zygote, 16–17

ABOUT THE AUTHORS

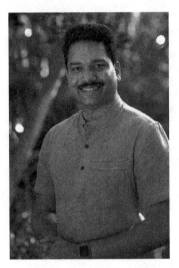

Vaidya Jayarajan Kodikannath is an internationally renowned Ayurvedic scholar, educator, author, and keynote speaker with over two decades of Ayurvedic clinical experience in India and the United States. Dr. J, as his students call him, is the chief executive officer and chief Ayurveda consultant of Kerala Ayurveda USA and president of the National Ayurvedic Medical Association (USA). He is a compassionate healer and educator devoted to propagating consciousness-based traditional teachings and practice of Ayurveda across the globe. He lives and practices in the San Francisco Bay Area with his wife and son.

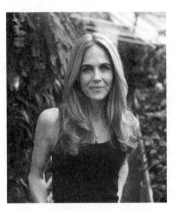

Alyson Young Gregory is a parenting media writer specializing in holistic health, a certified Ayurvedic health counselor and educator, and a registered yoga teacher (E-RYT) with Yoga Alliance. She is originally from New York, where she studied with the founders of the Nosara Yoga Institute and taught children's yoga and meditation. She completed her Ayurvedic studies with Vaidya Jayarajan Kodikannath at Kerala Ayurveda USA, where she is an alumna and works as part of a full-spectrum global organization with deep roots in India, committed to transforming healthcare science in the twenty-first century. She lives in the Boston area with her daughter.